STO

Y0-BST-905

5.16.'79

# REJUVENATION

*Books by Linda Clark*

Stay Young Longer
Get Well Naturally
Secrets of Health and Beauty
Help Yourself to Health (an ESP book)
Know Your Nutrition
Be Slim AND Healthy
Face Improvement through
    Exercise and Nutrition
Are You Radioactive? (How·to Protect Yourself)
The Best of Linda Clark (an anthology)
Color Therapy
Health, Youth and Beauty Through
    Color Breathing (with Yvonne Martine)
Beauty Questions and Answers (with Karen Kelly)
The Linda Clark Cookbook
A Handbook of Natural Remedies for Common Ailments
Rejuvenation
The Health and Beauty Book for Pets:
    A Nutritional Guide
How to Improve Your Health:
    The Wholistic Approach

*To find any of these books please inquire at your health store, bookstore, or library. Most of them are available in paperback.*

LINDA
CLARK

# REJUVENATION

THE DEVIN-ADAIR COMPANY
Old Greenwich

Library of Congress Catalog Card Number: 77-92696
ISBN: 0-8159-6718-7

Printed in the United States of America

# CONTENTS

# Publisher's Preface

Does growing older mean inevitably "getting old"? Linda Clark, America's top health and nutrition reporter, declares it need not be so. It is possible to maintain vigor and mental alertness into advanced years by natural means available to everyone — and by a positive resolution "to be the person you want to be," whatever your age. In this her fifteenth book she shows explicitly and clearly how to retard and even reverse the gradual deterioration of the body's mechanism we take for granted as "normal" to the process of aging. Her rejuvenation program is based on long investigation and study of the causes of such deterioration and effective measures for preventing it. Those measures represent tested and proven findings of renowned scientists and recognized experts in the field and include developments so recent, as well as remarkable, that news of them appears in this book for the first time in any publication.

Linda Clark dismisses the dream of a quick miracle-cure, a mythical Fountain of Youth. What she offers instead are ways within the range of everyone, which, when adopted and followed regularly, enable the body to restore itself and remain in a healthy state indefinitely.

Contrary to longstanding belief, seemingly aging cells can be regenerated and poorly functioning glands reactivated if supplied the nutrients and supplements they lack. She tells us exactly what they are, explains the purpose of each, explains how to use them, lists where to obtain them.

Above all, she provides guidelines for restructuring habits and lifestyles on all levels that have contributed to the debilitation associated with aging. It is not only what we take in to rebuild the organism that counts, but also stimulating its distribution to where in the body it is needed. To bring this about both exercise and proper breathing are essential. For those who frown at the mention of exercise Linda Clark has assembled an assortment of simple routines from which to choose, each of them demanding little time or effort, yet which do the job and can also be fun.

On another level, appearance can play a major role in staying fit as the years pile up. Looking your best at any age improves your self-image and how others see you. You do not have to spend a minor fortune going to beauty spas and plastic surgeons. There are reasonably priced — and absolutely safe — products you can use with results that perform near miracles.

And finally, but far from least, is mental attitude. Though age admittedly brings its special problems and often misfortunes, there is no reason to let them be defeating. You can change your life through thought, as is demonstrated by case histories and some practical, commonsense suggestions that make it less hard to do than it may seem at times.

*Rejuvenation* has been eagerly awaited by a large audience of health-minded readers, and by many more who realize that the day to become health-minded can no longer be postponed. They will not be disappointed. For this is undoubtedly and will long remain the definitive book on the prevention of aging. No one over forty will want to miss it. No one under forty can fail to benefit from it in preparing for the years ahead.

*—Florence Norton*

## A Note to the Reader

Due to an overcrowded schedule and an increasing number of letters and requests for information, Linda Clark cannot correspond with readers. She is not legally allowed to prescribe, recommend, or advise on individual health problems, nor to mention brand names in correspondence. As a reporter, however, she can report on research and direct you to the information you need. For further details about your questions, see Postscript, page 191.

# 1

## Aging Can Be Pleasant

THIS MORNING I received a phone call from one of my daughters. She lives in New York, I live in California. She apologized when I answered the phone. "I'm sorry to bother you with a problem, Mom," she began, "But I am at my wits' end with one of my teen-age children. I need suggestions and advice." She then outlined the problem.

I felt flattered to receive this call because most younger parents these days are contemptuous about advice from their elders. They want to do things *their* way without any interference from the older generation, who are too often considered old fogies. Believe me, I have learned the hard way, that it is not wise to offer advice unless it is asked for, otherwise it will be rejected. But in this case it was asked for, and since my daughter knew I had at one time been a teen-age counselor as well as a parent, she hoped I would know the solution. Fortunately, I had an answer that satisfied her and relieved her worry.

Before this phone call I had already been at work on

this book, inspired by my discovery that the older generation in the United States has become a forgotten species. Whereas in their younger years they were active, admired by others, fresh and vital in appearance, as the years have rolled by these same people find that they are becoming "has-beens," too often ignored, and left on the shelf in loneliness or illness and with nothing pleasant to look forward to.

Most of us Seniors, of which I am now one, have had our heyday. As an international lecturer and writer I have had my share of attention on the platform, radio, and TV. I have been a consultant, as I explained, to teen-agers, and later to middle-agers. One day not too long ago I was with my second daughter when we met a stranger who knew nothing about either of us. The not-too-young stranger, a man, could not take his eyes off my daughter, who is admittedly attractive, while he ignored me completely, the first time this had ever happened. So I know how it feels. Please understand: I did not begrudge the attention to my daughter, who is both lovely and lovely looking, but I did begrudge the fact that the newcomer did not even acknowledge that I existed.

I suddenly realized what a Senior has to face. Many are considered burdens by their children, who do not know what to do with them. Retirement homes or centers are a help, but even they can be depressing because of so many old, decrepit people present, leaning on canes, walking on crutches, or pushing about in wheelchairs. And the average nursing home is usually worse.

Some people, as they get older, are in better condition than others. We have all seen pictures in the newspapers of centenarians or couples who have celebrated their fiftieth or sixtieth anniversary. And they look it! You think, "But for the grace of God, there go I!" But others at late ages are alert, vital, healthy, and really enjoying life. I know a counselor in her eighties who never forgets anything, is in constant demand by people all over the nation. Her phone is never idle. Another couple, about ninety, an elderly retired doctor and his wife (he has long been interested in reversing aging), have a ten-acre ranch they supervise, and they love every minute of it. Others are adored by their children and friends and are sought after, admired, and respected by people of various ages.

There are people in different parts of the world who live to, and well beyond, the hundred-year mark, enjoying good vision, hearing, health, and tremendous endurance all the way. Men at this late age even beget children. These Seniors are in far better condition than some of our American forty- and fifty-year-olds. They are also respected for their wisdom, consulted by their juniors, and, in short, lead happy, useful lives.[1,2,3] This is as it should be.

Several researchers in the field of gerontology (fancy name for the study of aging) insist that the human body, if treated right, is good for at least a hundred years of active, enjoyable, healthy life. So being older does not necessarily mean we need be decrepit.

Fortunately, forced retirement at age sixty-five is on its way out. Some states have already reversed the ruling. Undoubtedly, others will soon follow. The stigma of mandatory retirement at sixty-five is limiting to the individual and to society. For too long public policy has been influenced by a person's number of years

rather than by ability. The woman counselor previously mentioned, who is extremely successful and praised
for her helpful services to clients, told me recently that
although she is in her eighties, she dare not say so or
her clients would lose confidence in her because of her
age and she might lose her job. This is absurd.

Age sixty-five, and beyond, should not be the end of
life, but, as with those in their forties and fifties, just
the beginning!

Meanwhile, too many identify aging with wrinkles, a
tottery gait, and general disability. This need not be so
either. Instead of cringing as we get older, we should
learn how to rehabilitate ourselves so that we can be
proud to be good examples of an age at which we have
earned the respect of everyone.

So the number of years one lives should not be the
criterion of ability during so-called aging. If we make it
so, it is our own fault. We should refuse to give in to
the aging process and should begin to do something
constructive about it so that we get better as we get
older, not worse.

We all want to be needed, loved, and respected by
others instead of being shelved. That is why I was flattered to receive the phone call from my daughter mentioned at the beginning.

For many months I have been searching widely for
methods of rehabilitation or prevention of so-called
aging problems. I have tried them all personally, and
those that have proved successful in personal improvement I will share with you in this book.

To begin with, I do not like to be called a "senior citizen" or, even worse, "elderly." Such pity-evoking
terms are but further stigmas in our American way of

life. I prefer the term "Senior." Seniors in high school
are looked up to; Seniors in college are looked up to by
other undergraduates. Why not Seniors in life? So let's
begin our rehabilitation by using this term. Don't think
of yourself as elderly or a senior citizen, but as a respected *Senior*. In fact, do not tell your age at all unless you want to or have to. Some people advertise
their advancing years with pride, hoping to attract
sympathy or hoping that people will exclaim, "Surely
you can't be *that* old!" I know one ninety-four-year-
old woman who looks closer to the average sixty-four.
She is slim, trim, attractive, chic, and well groomed.
She has good eyesight, good hearing, good health, and
is mentally alert. She is incredible, but not vain about
it, accepting her condition as her due. She never tells
her age. Her relatives are the ones who are proud of
her.

Americans are criticized for being so concerned
about the perpetuation of youth that it amounts to a
craze. No wonder. Since most oldsters have allowed
themselves to become decrepit, no one wants to be
around them. I believe we must reverse the trend so
that younger people will really want to be with us. But
we must work to improve ourselves and earn respect
from others. Having finally become a Senior myself, I
realize that most Seniors need counseling the same as
teen-agers and middle-agers. And so I decided I want
to help bring credit to our group. I hope you will join
me.

Instead of becoming glued to TV or a rocking chair,
we should begin by getting off our fannies and doing
something commendable. One good start is to be of
service to others, *any* service you can find. If you have

certain knowledge at your disposal, dust it off and put it to use. If not, learn something new. Higher education is enjoying an unprecedented boom all over the United States. Colleges and universities are offering adult courses for those who want to earn a college degree without leaving their area, or who are giving up other activities, even jobs, for additional learning denied earlier. Many women who had to cut short their education due to marriage and having children now have a chance to complete their studies. Others are seeking, and getting, instruction for a new career or an enriched retirement. Courses in Shakespeare, history, psychology, art of various kinds, languages, law, calligraphy, even horseback riding are available.

You may say that you don't feel well enough to take up a new interest. This is a common complaint of Seniors and as such is the main subject of this book: *How to feel better as well as look better. It can be done.* But, again, no one but *you* can do it. Now is the time for you to get busy so that you will be ready for anything you would really like to do, yet hesitate to attempt because of your present condition. It is not necessary to sit around waiting for the grim reaper!

If you fear death, this too can be overcome. Some metaphysicians tell us that we die only when we are ready to die, not before, no matter what the circumstance of death. One man was killed by a falling tree. This was no accident (metaphysicians and parapsychologists do not believe there are "accidents"). The explanation given was that the man was ready to die and walked under the tree of his own volition when it was ready to fall. Some go still farther. They insist that we choose our time to be born, our parents, our birthplace and date, and the type of life we are to lead in order to learn the lessons we need to learn. I am not urging you to believe this, merely suggesting that there are those who have studied the subject in depth to learn that we have been given a free will to do whatever we wish. According to this philosophy, you make your own life and cannot blame circumstances, your parents, your children, or anyone else for the results. Remember this point, since it bears on what kind of life you can build for yourself so that you *will* like it!

Some people do not fear death as much as the moment of dying, which they believe involves great pain. We are told that this is not necessarily so: The spirit, or soul, is apparently lifted free of the body before actual death takes place. The impact of a car, plane, or other accident is not felt.

How do we know this? Because some people have died, and returned to tell us about the experience. Surprisingly, these reports agree. There are stories galore of people who have "died" on the operating table or by other means. The returnee has stated that life on the other side is beautiful, painless, and like walking into "God's other room," filled with beautiful flowers, music, scenery, as well as friends, relatives, and other loved ones, even pets, who have preceded them. The reason they returned, they stated, is that they were sent back because their job here was not yet finished or someone needed them. They did return, but because of the experience they lost all fear of death once and for all.

Dr. Elisabeth Kübler-Ross, formerly a country doctor in Switzerland, now a Chicago psychiatrist and author and lecturer, specializes in helping people conquer the fear of dying. In an interview published in the *San Francisco Chronicle*, December 5, 1975, she told of her research, which has convinced her that "beyond a shadow of a doubt" there is life after death. She tells of accident victims doctors thought had died, but who later revived. These patients said they had a feeling of departing from their physical bodies and floating blissfully above them, even hearing everything said by the doctors and nurses, which was later confirmed.[4]

Dr. Kübler-Ross tells of a two-year-old boy who apparently died, but was later saved by doctors. He told his mother he was dead and it was so beautiful where he went that he did not want to come back; he added that he was with Mary and Jesus. But Mary told him he must go back to help his mother.

More such case histories are listed in the best-selling book, *Life After Life*, by Raymond A. Moody, Jr., M.D.

So, rather than spending time and energy worrying about dying, you can postpone the date of dying and spend the same time and energy in making your life pleasant until you are ready to go. Since you have been given a free will, you can use it for good or bad, happiness or sadness. You can be the person you want to be. You can be vital, flexible, healthy, attractive, alert, and happy *at any age*. You can program such a life and make it yours!

Or, if you insist, you can do the opposite. You can be negative, complaining, critical, full of self-pity and unhappiness, attracting negative people and conditions into your life. Nobody will stop you if that's what you want.

Your life is what you make it. You, and you alone, are the pilot, and you can compute how you are going to spend the remaining years of your life. You have heard the statement: "Today is the beginning of the rest of your life." You need not live in the past, repeating to bored listeners what has already happened to you. You can embark on a new life and a happy, healthy existence.

It can be done. It has been done. This book will tell you how to do it. Be prepared for some fascinating surprises to help you on your way!

### REFERENCES
(See *Bibliography* for fuller details)

1. Bernard Jensen, *World Keys to Health and Long Life.*
2. Sula Benet, *How to Live to Be 100.*
3. Grace Halsell, *Los Viejos, Secrets of Long Life from the Sacred Valley.*
4. Elisabeth Kübler-Ross, M.D., *On Death and Dying.*
      ———, *Death, The Final Stage of Growth.*
5. Raymond A. Moody, Jr., M.D., *Life After Life.*

# 2

## Why Your Body Needs Help

WE TAKE OUR bodies and health for granted—at first. As long as they work reasonably well and don't give us any trouble, we pay little attention to them. But when they begin to complain and stop working properly, with small disturbances like headaches and constant colds and later more serious ailments, then we panic and are ready to stop the neglect and do something about it. We have had a rude awakening to the fact our bodies and health are not necessarily automatic.

When we were born, we didn't realize what a gold mine we had. Unless during pregnancy our mother took drugs, smoked excessively, was an alcoholic, or did not eat right, we were probably born with good health and all the necessary parts. Otherwise we may have been marked at birth with a defect or diseased condition. Some babies, born of alcoholic mothers, actually come into this world with alcohol on their breath like a drunken adult. Or if the nutrition of the mother lacked a certain vitamin at a specific time during pregnancy, the child could be born with a cleft palate. This has been definitely established in many cases.

Even heart defects, eyes that need glasses early in life, and a host of other "inherited" weaknesses are often due to the fact that the mother did not eat the right food during pregnancy to provide her child with the correct building material. If she added drugs or other poisons, the baby paid additionally for it throughout its lifetime.

What about the statement that to be in good health we should choose our ancestors? This can be true because of our genes, those mysterious inborn influences that affect our bodies, our appearance, our behavior, and our health. These genes may be inherited from our parents, grandparents, and great-grandparents. Not only do different families have certain genes; certain nationalities do too. Orientals can eat and thrive on food Americans may or may not thrive on. Italians, Norwegians, and other nationalities, ditto. This does not mean that Americans cannot enjoy Oriental or Italian food occasionally. But for a steady diet the people of one country may not thrive on the full-time diet of another country. For example, the amount of protein available for one country may not satisfy the needs of another. The Norwegians thrive on fish, which is plentiful in that area. The Italians for the most part keep their figures eating pasta every day, whereas Americans who are overly fond of spaghetti are apt to be fat. Various peoples have been conditioned for centuries by the genes of their own nationality. The body does not welcome sudden, sharp changes, and it may take a generation or more to adjust to such changes.

Our glands, the machines that run our bodies, are also affected by our ancestors. If they ate good, wholesome food, this served as good "fuel" for their glands, which were passed on to their children and

their successors. But if the good fuel was not constantly supplied, the glands of one generation could fail to
protect them, or the next generation.

I have already told the story elsewhere of four children, a sister and three brothers, who lived to ripe old
ages with surprisingly good health in spite of a poor
diet. On searching further, I learned that the parents of
these four children lived on a farm, as did their parents, and *their* parents. Their food was nutritious, their
health was good. Glands were sustained by wholesome farm food, and health was evident in each generation—up until the final one, the woman and her three
brothers. *They had moved to a city and eaten city food.*
Even so, they lived to an incredibly advanced age until
suddenly, one by one, each of them "fell apart" and
died. It was similar to a house that looks sound on the
outside, then one day collapses from termites that
have been riddling the inside of the structure. The
poor city diet had caught up with this family. Good
glands could not be perpetuated without proper fuel,
so they finally gave out.

When we are born, let us hope with a healthy body,
we have a possession money can't buy. Our parents, if
they are wise, take care of our bodies for us until we
are old enough and presumably wise enough to assume
that responsibility. But at this point most people begin
to deteriorate without realizing it. They eat what tastes
good, ignoring whether or not it is good for them. They
begin to smoke, drink, and take drugs because it is the
"thing" to do. They lose sleep, burn the candle at both
ends, and resent it if anyone tells them not to. They
start gaining weight on junk food and then try to take it
off with a fad diet that leaves their bodies even more

nutritionally exhausted. They begin to develop aches and pains, and rush to the nearest doctor to patch them up with drugs. Unfortunately, drugs do not cure; they merely give temporary relief, as, for example, an aspirin may stop a headache but it does not remove the cause.

So not until the body starts to scream do we become scared. The aches and pains are the forerunners of old age. Yet if you warn young people to stop taking their most precious assets—their body and health—for granted and urge them to start treating these assets with respect, they rebel at "authority." You probably did the same thing yourself. We all learn the hard way, or else we do not know what to do the right way.

Dr. José Froimovich, a distinguished gerontologist from Chile, who has devoted over thirty-five years to the study of the causes of aging, says: "Deterioration of our body is a result of increasing deficiencies within the body's tissue. Yet such conditions can be changed." He continues: "Why should we accept as an unchangeable fact of life that our body should start to give out just when life's experience enables our brain to function at its best? This very period in our life is the most valuable age for the human in society."

Fortunately, it is possible to reprogram our glands and to reverse many of these aging symptoms, if you know how. And that is what this book is about.

You will find many helps in this book. You may not be able to follow them all. If you cannot, there is no need to feel guilty. Make note of those that appeal to you as you read the book, jot them down in the empty pages at the back of the book with the correct page number, and gradually include as many as you can.

# 3

## The Effect of Cells
## on Rejuvenation

OUR BODIES are made of cells, or to turn it around, cells help make our bodies. They occur in all tissues, including the skin, every muscle, every gland, every organ. They are the foundation of the body structure. I am not punning when I say never sell a cell short. Nurture your cells, encourage them, pamper them, and you will be paid back in full with accrued interest.

Because your cells are the fabric from which your body is woven, with proper care you can help your cells prevent your body from wearing out prematurely. When your car wears out, you must buy a new one. When your body wears out, you cannot buy a new one, but you can help your cells rehabilitate the body you already have.

There are about sixty trillion cells in the body, a number impossible to visualize. They age at different rates in different ways. But the slowdown of the creation of new cells is the basis of aging. This cell loss is greater in the glands, nerves, muscles, and kidneys. Cell loss can also be due at any age to poisons in the environment, such as air pollution, or to alcohol, smoking, radiation, even some food additives. Certain vitamins (C and E) can help protect the cells from such disturbances.[1]

Cells are constantly dying and being replaced with new cells. In early youth newly formed cells outnumber the dying cells. In middle age the number of dying cells is balanced by equivalent new cells. In aging the old cells may die faster than they can be replaced by new cells. Old cells divide to form new cells, but old cells that have gone through many divisions are less efficient in division and rebirth. Some scientists believe that certain cells, such as brain cells, do not divide at all. So we must protect the cells we already have.

Hans J. Kugler, Ph.D., the author of a book on slowing down the aging process, states: "It is therefore of the most importance to supply our cells with optimum conditions *at all times* in order to keep them alive for the longest time possible."[2]

The body is said to renew itself completely every seven years, but the quality of the new cells can be no better, as the cell manufacture continues, than the material, or food, on which they are fed. If the cells are allowed to deteriorate, they may reproduce inferior offspring—cells of poor quality, which in turn are perpetuated. As you can see, this creates second-, third-, or fourth-class cells incapable of keeping the body functioning at top performance.

But there is still hope when this happens. Other scientists have learned that at certain stages, if only 10 per cent of the cells are in good condition, with the proper help those cells can eventually regenerate the entire body. Cell reproduction in early youth is rapid and automatic, whereas it may take longer for cells to regenerate toward the later years in life. So we cannot leave it to chance; we must work at it!

Even so, there is proof that, given the proper conditions, cells can multiply faster than usual. In the Department of Molecular, Cellular, and Developmental Biology, University of Colorado, researchers found that cells growing in laboratory flasks could be reconstructed within a span of several hours. The researchers found that they could take cells apart and put them together again in better combinations than before. This discovery surprised even the team of scientists who accomplished this feat.[3] In 1975 two research physiologists at the University of California, Drs. Lester Packer and James R. Smith, found that by raising the oxygen level in cells and exposing the cells to visible light, the treated cells continued to grow and reproduce beyond the 120-division point, comparable to more than double their usual life span.

And there is still earlier proof in a well-known example. In 1912 Dr. Alexis Carrel initiated an experiment at the Rockefeller Institute for Medical Research in New York. He placed a fraction of heart muscle in a nutrient medium, and this piece of heart muscle lived for over thirty years, at which time the experiment was discontinued. Dr. Carrel received a Nobel Prize for his achievement. *But certain nutrients were needed to feed and nourish the heart muscle in order to keep it alive and well.*[4]

Other similar, more recent, experiments are in progress. As proof, at Lawrence Berkeley Laboratory, cells assumed to reproduce only fifty times divided 120 times, and are still dividing. Vitamin E is used as a nutrient, and the cells appear young and healthy.[5] But additional nutrients are also needed.

Dr. José Froimovich, mentioned in the previous chapter, has supplied certain nutrients to scores of aging men and women and has produced amazing results in their rehabilitation, about which more later. It is interesting to note at this point that Dr. Froimovich believes we are not living to our full age potential of 100 to 120 years. Yet there are scores of examples of members of various groups in Europe and elsewhere who do live that long and in good health, as we have already learned. But in these cases certain requirements have been fulfilled for them during their entire lives. One of the requirements appears to be correct food; another, sufficient oxygen. Both are needed for optimum health and survival of the cells.

Man cannot live without oxygen. We can live for some time without food, less time without water, but we can survive only a few minutes without oxygen. Normally we get our oxygen from the air. Today, unfortunately, because of air pollution the oxygen supply is affected, interfering with the amount delivered to the cells of those who breathe contaminated air. Even if the body takes in sufficient air, in some people the oxygen necessary to sustain certain parts of the body cannot adequately reach these areas to provide proper nourishment, and the cells suffer. This is especially true of the brain, eyes, ears, and heart, which can become oxygen-starved, resulting in malfunction. Have you noticed how many people suffer from fuzzy thinking? They start to tell you something, perhaps about somebody, and cannot remember the point or recall the name of the person. Put it down to too little oxygen supply! It is becoming a common occurrence for all ages.

Fortunately, there are methods of providing oxygen and proper nourishment not only to stimulate cells and glands, but also to remove waste products, thus renewing both cells and glandular functions. This, in turn, helps to slow down or reverse the aging process and encourages the body to rehabilitate itself. This is a new and exciting concept, and I will tell you how to do it in a later chapter.

In some hospitals there are now oxygen machines for out-patients. The wife of one man, who was depressed and could not remember anything well, told me that after a short treatment by one of these machines the temporary change in his behavior and mental acuity was almost unbelievable. Someone else has suggested that the time may come (if air contamination continues) when we may rent or buy an oxygen machine for home use to provide us with a dose when we need it. Other, easier methods of increasing our oxygen supply will be discussed subsequently.

Certain nutrients can stimulate the oxygen supply in various cells of the body. This should not be confused with cell therapy, popular in Europe and discussed in chapter 10, by which fresh animal cells are injected into waning bodies. People I have talked to who have had this therapy have mixed feelings about the results. In some cases, they report, the process did provide temporary vitality, in some instances more, in others less, but the effect often was of limited duration. Apparently cell nutrients are needed on a *continuous basis*. This you can achieve in your own home.

But this places the responsibility fully upon your own shoulders. You, all on your own, can help control your health and prevent rapid aging. No one else can do it for you. Your life is in your own hands, and it is never too late to begin to attain improvement. The sooner you start, the earlier the results.

### REFERENCES
(See *Bibliography* for fuller details)

1. Richard A. Passwater, *Supernutrition.*
2. Hans J. Kugler, *Slowing Down the Aging Process.*
   ———, *Seven Keys to a Longer Life.*
3. *Proceedings of the National Academy of Science,* May, 1974.
4. Ivan Popov, M.D., *Stay Young.*
5. Richard A. Passwater, *Supernutrition for Healthy Hearts.*

# 4

## Wake Up
## Your Glands

THE GLANDS in your body are some of the most important machinery you own. They control vital functions that influence your health as well as the rate of aging. For years prophets of doom have been warning us that after the age of forty our glands begin to slow down, and there is nothing we can do about it. To that statement I say "Bosh!"

If this is so, why is it that there are those, regardless of age, who are as mentally alert as a much younger person? Why is it that in some parts of the world men and women live to the ripe age of a hundred and beyond? Why is it that men at this late date have retained their sexual potency and even sired children? It is undoubtedly because the glands of these people are still in good working order. If some people can keep their glands in good condition, why not you?

Glands, as well as cells, need proper fuel, which is absolutely essential to keep them in good condition. It is no doubt true that genes (which you inherit from your ancestors) also play a part. But how did your ancestors' glands become so superior? Their way of life, as well as proper fuel, had a decided effect. Even if you have inherited or developed poor glands, researchers say they can be improved. The proper fuel (nutrition), plus exercise, plus the right mental attitude can combine to help bring about this improvement.

In younger years glands and cells seem to function almost automatically. Youngsters usually do not give it all a second thought. They appear to have inexhaustible energy and usually look well regardless of what they eat or do. However, if they live on junk food, dissipate, ignore sleep, good hygiene, exercise, and other body-caring measures, little by little their glandular machinery is sabotaged. A kind of time bomb slowly builds up as the continual use of poor fuel, drugs, alcohol, smoking, and other such indignities undermines the health and strength of the precious glands. Toxins accumulate in the body, and your once seemingly foolproof body or machine now suddenly develops knocks, creaks, and groans. With alarm you begin to think, "I'm getting old!"

There is nothing unexplainable or even sudden about what has happened. Your gradual mistreatment of your body has been going on for a long time until finally the time bomb does explode. But this, of all times, is not the moment to give up. Instead, you will have to switch the control from automatic to manual and take over your own programming. This is the moment to get busy.

I am told by people who work in nursing and retirement homes that many who live there have given up and lost the will to live. They are anxious to die and get the misery over with. Otherwise they might not be there at all. If they were full of pep, enjoying life, attractive to others, no one would force them, or even want them, to be there. In Europe and in the East particularly, older men and women are respected for their wisdom and other assets. They remain with their families, who love and enjoy them and want them in their home circle as long as they live.

But since you yourself have produced this condition of so-called "aging," which is actually little more than prolonged neglect, you can also dig yourself out and pull yourself up by your own bootstraps. The information on how to do it is fascinating and included in this book. Roll up your sleeves and get to work. You will find information to help you look better within minutes. You will find information to help you feel better and more energetic within a few short months. But *this means adopting a completely new way of life from now on.* Once you decide to rehabilitate yourself, you must not turn back. Is it worth the effort? You bet it is. You will not only find something to live for, but this new way of life will help you to enjoy life more than ever before.

A program to get you started on your way will show you, first, what to eat, later, how to exercise pleasantly and easily, and still later, how to think your way to rejuvenation.

Others have accomplished wonders. So can you.

### *Tips for Success*

1. Get a large notebook, or use the empty pages at the back of this book. Write down the items you wish to incorporate in your programs as you read about them

or think of them. You may have to adjust the program to your own needs.

2. Read what you have written every day so you will not forget.

3. *Do not talk about this program to others.* Otherwise they may try to discourage you. Remember that when someone announces embarking on a reducing diet, for some reason almost everyone tries to interfere and tempt the would-be reducer to abandon the program. So do not talk about this program, just do it quietly and firmly.

4. You may, at first, notice only a good day now and then. These occasional good days may be followed by one or more bad days. The reason? The body does not like change. It likes the old routine, the old comfort. But this program will have to be *a new way of life.* As you are consistent, eventually the good days will outnumber the bad days. One expert who has observed the effects of this program on many people says it usually takes from one to three months (depending on how far gone you were when you started) before you realize you are feeling really good. Whatever happens, *don't give up.* Eventually, first one reward, then another will become evident

5. There is no quick panacea, no magic wand, no single secret (except determination and work) to produce a miracle when your back is turned. Results come from an applied program of combined approaches, both mental and physical.

Are you ready? If so, I am ready to turn over the keys to you. Good luck.

# 5

# New vs. Old
# Medical Treatment

THE BELIEFS that people are staying young longer and that Americans are the healthiest people in the world are myths. The United States is close to the bottom of the list, both in longevity and health, and if you believe people here stay young longer, just visit any hospital for the aged or nursing home, all of which are crowded with unhealthy, unhappy, aged people.

As for living longer, Richard A. Passwater states in his book *Supernutrition*: "Contrary to popular belief, neither the maximum life-span nor the age of death for people living past the age of twenty has increased significantly since 1800." It may be true that *some* people are staying young longer, are healthier than usual in later age, but these people are exceptions. Either their genes are special, or they have learned what to do to help themselves, as this book is intended to help *you*.

There are basically two types of disease: infectious and degenerative. Infectious diseases are those that are usually contagious and are transmitted by a "germ" from other people, food, water, air, insects, soil, and other sources. A cold, flu, smallpox, malaria, amoebic dysentery, even tuberculosis are all considered infectious diseases. Infectious disease *may* respond to a drug, depending on the disease, but the drug must be chosen carefully by the doctor, since some drugs produce side effects worse than the disease itself. In a life-or-death matter an antibiotic or so-called "miracle drug" may indeed save a life. But these drugs should not be used indiscriminately or continued indefinitely. For routine ailments there are safer and wiser treatments.

I recently learned of two doctors who found this out for themselves. One doctor was caught in a blizzard on a house call to the back country, where, abandoning his car, he nearly collapsed as he was forced to reach safety on foot. He fell, breaking several ribs, and was rescued by a farmer's family, who gave him not only shelter but every type of home care: good food, a comfortable bed, and tender loving attention. Since his "black bag" had been left behind in his car, there were no drugs available. He gave his rescuers instructions for strapping his ribs correctly. There was nothing else to do but wait for the road plow to get through and bring medical help. This took nearly two weeks while the doctor was recuperating from shock, stress, and pain.

Eventually another doctor arrived, complete with drugs. But the injured doctor refused the drugs. He said to the surprised visiting doctor: "I am astonished how, without any drugs at all, I have been getting well anyway. I have given this much thought and have decided I have been overdoing drugs with my patients. I am going to stop it!''

Let's face it, Nature knows better than man. There are other types of healing remedies that are more natural and effective and safer than drugs. For example, vitamin C, if used in proper amounts, has cured infections after a drug has proved useless. Homeopathy is another type of medical treatment elected by a few doctors after they have completed their medical school training. Many homeopathic physicians have become so amazed at the quick, easy, and effective recoveries from a myriad of diseases that they have largely given up the use of drugs. The tiny homeopathic tablets, used for centuries with safety, are chosen with great care for the *person*, not the *disease*, and have produced miracle after miracle in healing when drugs have failed. Orthodox doctors condemn them as "folly," even though the doctors who use homeopathy have had the same initial medical training and have merely added homeopathy as an extra elective upon their graduation.[1] Many orthodox doctors, who do not understand this type of treatment, laugh at it. They also laugh at nutrition for the same reason.

Yet some open-minded doctors are beginning to study and use not only homeopathy, but such alternative therapies as nutrition, herbs, acupuncture or acupressure (without needles), even spiritual healing, with remarkable success. And the nutritional approach to disease is sweeping the world as a result of patients who have tried these safer, simpler remedies with astonishing results.[2]

It is heartwarming that some doctors are beginning

to turn to these more natural methods, alternatives to routine use of drugs. A recent convention called "The Physician of the Future" was attended by seventy-two doctors. The event, featuring such alternatives, proved so successful that it was repeated the following year with 2,500 doctors present! The program also included the study of nutrition (vitamins and minerals, etc.), which doctors are not taught in medical schools, but which patients are demanding. As a result, many flexible doctors are beginning to study and learn on their own this logical nutritional method of helping their patients. An era of medical freedom is apparently in sight.

Degenerative diseases are a different problem altogether from infectious diseases. These include cardiovascular disease, arteriosclerosis or atherosclerosis, high blood pressure, diabetes, hypoglycemia, kidney diseases, some types of arthritis, and others. Such diseases involve a breakdown of body cells, eventually leading to the degeneration of the body itself. Drugs may temporarily remove some of the *symptoms,* but do not remove the cause. We have noted how aspirin stops a headache, but does not remove the underlying cause. Scientists and some doctors are just beginning to realize that a degenerative disturbance or disease can actually be due to undernutrition, causing the breakdown of the cells that have not been fed properly and leading to various degenerative diseases in various people, depending upon individual weaknesses. As proof, many times these degenerative conditions have been reversed by restoring the deficiency through proper nutrition.

Meanwhile, a great many orthodox doctors refuse to

accept this concept, since they were taught about drugs only. They really believe that the nutritional approach is fraudulent. An example of this comes to mind. Recently, after finding that natural food fiber in the diet (rather than bland, unnatural foods) could prevent many intestinal ailments, including cancer, doctors the world over were electrified at the news. The physicians who had made the discovery took X-rays and photographs of African natives on both types of diet and showed these pictures to international medical groups. A doctor in one group that viewed these convincing pictures was heard to say, "I cannot believe my eyes that anything you put in your mouth could improve your health."

This shocking statement indicates that the lack of nutritional instruction in medical school amounts to brainwashing. As another example, at a hearing against a nutritional M.D. who has been getting people well by nutrition instead of drugs, and therefore provoking the wrath of the orthodox medics, who persecuted him and took away his license, it became clear that the accusing orthodox doctors present actually sincerely believed that nutrition as medicine is a fraud. Even transplants of heart, kidney, and other organs (with a high death rate) are being used instead of the easier, safer, painless, and natural remedies. Again we come to the superiority of nature as compared with the ineffectuality of man. For instance, everyone has heard of patients who have received a clean bill of health following a medical checkup and who died from a heart attack within days or weeks.[3]

In the case of degenerative disease, feeding the cells and glands what they need has helped many to become and remain stronger, thus preventing (or reversing) degeneration. This method has even benefited some infectious diseases through prevention, since proper nutrition can help the body build more resistance to both bacterial and viral invasions.

In the next chapter you will see how nutrition can be an important factor in conquering degenerative diseases that, to date, have been considered killers. Be prepared for some encouraging surprises. This method provides great hope.

REFERENCES
(See *Bibliography* for fuller details)

1. Due to orthodox pressures very few homeopaths are available. For a free list of them and their addresses write: The National Center for Homeopathy, 6231 Leesburg Pike, Falls Church, Virginia 22044.
2. Linda Clark, *How to Improve Your Health: The Wholistic Approach.*
3. Wayne Martin, *Medical Heroes and Heretics.*

# 6

# What to Do About Degenerative Diseases

MANY SENIORS, as they become older, worry about the degenerative diseases from which so many of their friends or relatives die, especially heart attacks and strokes. Most of these premature deaths can be prevented by the newer, natural treatment: nutrition. Countless couples in their later years have been broken up by deaths from these ailments, leaving grieving widows or widowers to finish their lives alone. Treatments are now available to help prevent such unnecessary loss.

Furthermore, these treatments, tested and recommended by enlightened doctors, can usually be used at home. Since there is a saying, "You are as young as your arteries," which some people believe to be true, let us begin with arteries and how you can improve them.

### Artery Problems

Artery problems are usually classified as *arterio*sclerosis, and *athero*sclerosis. Their meaning differs slightly. *Arterio*sclerosis, often called hardening of the arteries, is actually a thickening and narrowing of the artery walls. *Athero*sclerosis, on the other hand, is a filling up or clogging of the arteries. As the clogging increases, the amount of blood that can be pumped through them diminishes, and various parts of the body, including the brain, eyes, arms, legs, or heart, may be cut off from their necessary blood supply, leading to strokes or heart attacks. Some people suffer from artery problems that are less serious, at least at first. So it is important to prevent or reverse this constriction of blood flow to all parts of the body. A book, *Live Longer Now*,[1] written by a group from the Longevity Research Institute of Santa Barbara, California, says: "Deposits in the arteries are called plaques, and these accumulate, perhaps leading to a complete block in the artery, or breaking into fragments. These fragments may be carried away in the bloodstream only to block another smaller artery some place downstream."

Fortunately, there are two ways to avoid this by natural methods. *Live Longer Now* gives one clue: "To live and do its job, each of the body's millions of cells needs to have nutrients brought to it by the blood supply . . . to keep the body cells alive and healthy, the arteries have to remain open and unclogged. If some of the arteries become clogged . . . the body cells served by those arteries will die *for lack of oxygen and other nutrients*" (emphasis added).

Too many people have artery problems without realizing it. But how can they avoid or reverse the condition? The treatment is twofold: (1) to provide the body with the correct nutrients to keep the cells healthy, as well as to dissolve the accumulations already present (this can be done and has been done); (2) to supply oxygen to the body cells for additional insurance and health. Natural, do-it-yourself techniques, discussed later, are available.

Orthodox physicians often resort to bypass surgery and drugs for artery problems. But the Longevity Research Institute (L.R.I.) has developed an alternative to these extreme therapies: They use a preventive program that consists mainly of a low-fat, low-cholesterol diet, plus exercise. To give this group due credit, this is definitely a step forward, at least compared to surgery and drugs; and by means of this program, the Institute has had some remarkable cases of patient improvement.

As an example, one woman had been treated for angina at age sixty-seven; for a severe heart attack at seventy-five; and still later, at eighty-one, for congestive heart failure, hypertension, angina, intermittent claudication, arthritis, and atherosclerosis. Finally she was placed on the Institute's program and, subsequently, won two gold medals in the 1974 California Senior Olympics. At eighty-five she has won four gold medals, runs a mile and a half daily, plus riding ten to fifteen miles on a stationary bicycle. She also does workouts at a gymnasium twice weekly.

This L.R.I. Program, which features the use of exercise, not only severely restricts cholesterol foods and fats, even many natural ones, but it also restricts vitamin/mineral supplements, considered so important by other researchers, who recommend these and other measures in addition to exercise with encouraging results.

## What Clogs Arteries?

In order to understand how you can unclog your arteries through natural methods, it is necessary to understand what clogs them. The deposits in the arteries have been found to be made up of fats, cholesterol, and sometimes calcium. Orthodox doctors assume that these substances *must* be present because they are taken in through the diet. Hence they warn their patients to stop eating cholesterol foods, such as organ meats (liver, sweetbreads, brains), even eggs and avocados, although these foods have some of the highest concentrations of vitamins, minerals, and hormones, all needed by the body and cells for health.

Nutritionists have denied for years that eggs and nutritious organ foods are dangerous. Now there is new, convincing evidence that they are right, and that there is a better way of handling the artery problem.[2]

Research shows that cholesterol is needed by the glands, including the sex glands, and if there is not enough of this substance available, the body manufactures it whether we eat it or not! In fact, a recent researcher stated that if we deny the body cholesterol in the form of foods, it works much more furiously to manufacture *more* cholesterol. So it appears that those who exclude these substances from the diet may be barking up a wrong tree.

Richard A. Passwater, whose specialties include the study of arteries as well as the subject of aging, reports in his book *Supernutrition* case after case of patients, including doctors, even heart specialists, who religiously avoided cholesterol foods and fat intake, but suffered a heart attack in spite of these measures.

Passwater observes: "Even though doctors have been warning us for fifty years that cholesterol . . . is the cause of atherosclerosis (deposits in the arteries) heart disease is striking increasingly larger portions of our population and at progressively earlier ages. . . . *If cholesterol reduction were effective, results would have been apparent long ago*" (emphasis added).

Dr. Passwater, a biochemist, admits that arteriosclerosis and atherosclerosis can be caused by cholesterol, fat, and certain calcium deposits, but, citing his proof, claims that reducing cholesterol intake not only does *not* reduce the deposits, but also does not reduce the cholesterol blood level or the onset of heart attacks. In fact, in his book he states that low cholesterol can *increase* the incidence of heart disease. He points out that research shows that earlier generations that ate gravies, fat meats, whole grains, and vegetables did not experience coronary thrombosis, so prevalent today.

Dr. Passwater points out that whole milk (not skim milk) and eggs are two of our best foods. He cites one study of 804,409 persons in which those who ate practically no eggs had more deaths from heart attacks and strokes than those who ate all the eggs they wanted.

What are the reasons behind these "scare tactics" against cholesterol and saturated fats? Brace yourself for an honest answer, as quoted in Dr. Passwater's book, from Dr. Teh C. Huang, a heart researcher: "Propaganda against cholesterol and saturated fat has been going on and been well accepted, while for centuries millions of human lives have been saved by milk and eggs. Don't cut out cholesterol and saturated fats from your diet. Warnings that they lead to heart disease are scare tactics by big business." ("Scare tactics" refers to high-profit sales of low cholesterol foods, including margarine.)

The highly nutritious natural foods, properly raised, contain natural vitamins and minerals. These foods are quite different from the highly processed foods that are so common today and from which vitamins and minerals have been removed. If any are returned to the food, they are fewer in number than those bestowed by nature, and they are usually synthetic, not natural. In addition, thousands of chemicals, colorings, fillers, and preservatives are added to foods to make them appear or taste more "natural." Even fresh garden produce or fruit may be less than nutritious, since much of this fresh food is polluted by pesticide sprays or contaminated by the highly chemicalized soil in which the food is grown, considered necessary by growers to stimulate faster growth and bigger crops. The few farmers and gardeners who grow their crops organically, which means that only natural fertilizers are used and nature controls the speed of growth, yielding a nutritious product instead of a hollow one, can't keep their produce long enough to supply all of their enthusiastic customers. Yet it is shocking that at this writing certain bureaucratic groups are attempting to ban the words "organic" and "natural" from labels even if the foods *are* organic and natural and therefore obviously more nutritious. Why? Because the big food processors apparently do not want such competition to the unnatural food they manufacture. You can usually tell the difference, because natural foods taste better. But the manufacturers are becoming more cunning with their masquerade and want us to believe their products are superior to natural ones.

Foods that are naturally endowed with vitamins and

minerals are not only preferable; there is much information that certain vitamins and minerals may protect
against heart attacks. This includes most minerals, as
well as vitamins E, C, B₆, and the entire B complex
family.

People who are afraid to eat *any* fat and adopt a
completely fat-free diet, either to avoid artery trouble
or for reducing purposes, can be piling up other troubles for themselves. Our bodies need fat for various
reasons. For example, a gall bladder denied fat can
produce gallstones.[3] Also, without fat in the diet, the
fat-soluble vitamins A, E, D, and K cannot be properly assimilated. Do not dismiss this problem lightly.
Without sufficient vitamin A your vision and skin can
suffer; without vitamin D, calcium, needed for bones,
is not properly assimilated. Without E the heart muscle can suffer, and without K blood clotting cannot occur, leading to hemorrhages.[4] So dietary fats are cru-
cially necessary.

Even those who avoid fat for fear of overweight
may be surprised to learn that it may be easier to reduce if some fat is eaten. Adelle Davis tells the story
of the model who could not lose weight until she added
a few tablespoons of vegetable oil to her daily diet.

### *How to Dissolve Artery Fat and Cholesterol*

THERE IS A WAY to emulsify or dissolve excess fat
and cholesterol deposits that may already have formed
in your arteries. It can also help prevent them. This
method was demonstrated by a physician, Lester M.
Morrison, M.D., author of *The Low-Fat Way to*

*Health and Longer Life.*[5]  This helpful book was written a number of years ago and generally ignored by physicians, although many nutritionists were aware of it. Adelle Davis used this method, in part, with great success to lower cholesterol levels in the blood. Since its publication additional nutritional information has become available, reported by others who recognize the effectiveness of the Morrison concept on artery problems.

Dr. Morrison learned that the substance lecithin (pronounced lessithin) is similar to a detergent taken orally and can dissolve or emulsify artery-plugging fats and cholesterol, even excess cholesterol in the blood. Dr. Morrison reported some dramatic results with his patients. They became able to walk again without difficulty if this had been a problem. They became more alert, vital, younger looking and acting in many cases. Even the yellowish plaques that had developed around their eyes were dissolved and disappeared. Dr. Morrison recommended four tablespoons of lecithin granules daily for his patients, to be taken in juices, on cereals, salads, or however convenient. Lecithin granules, made from soybeans, are somewhat nutty in texture but tasteless. Dr. Morrison, who was interested in nutrition, also advocated at least two tablespoons of soy or safflower oil daily to "provide the essential fatty acids necessary for proper nutrition." He recommended vitamins as well, especially B, C, and E. Meanwhile, though Dr. Morrison was ahead of his time with his discoveries about lecithin (additional exciting information will be discussed later), a newer type of lecithin has come on the market: liquid lecithin. Less of it is evidently necessary. One researcher found that one teaspoon taken morning and evening could keep it in the bloodstream at all times. It has been found to be effective in reversing some other difficult diseases too, including myasthenia gravis.[6]

Dr. William Donald Kelley recommends liquid lecithin, as did the late nutrition expert Dr. Royal Lee. Dr. Kelley recommends about one tablespoon of it daily and believes it is better than granular or powdered lecithin (another newcomer), because it contains, he says, a new unnamed vitamin missing in the other forms. Liquid lecithin is easier for some people to take, harder for others. It looks like honey, has the consistency of honey, but there the similarity ends. It tastes like nothing and sticks to a spoon as well as to the roof of your mouth.

There are two schools of thought on natural or preventive artery control. One school believes in sharply restricting fats and cholesterol foods, combined with exercise. This school of thought is represented by the Longevity Research Institute, discussed previously. A second school does not worry about fats and cholesterol foods but does emphasize vitamin/mineral supplements plus lecithin to prevent the possible nutritional deficiencies that may have caused the problem in the first place. This school of thought also embraces exercise. Reporters are not supposed to have opinions, but having been a nutrition reporter for many years, I must admit that, to me, the latter method makes sense and is the easier to follow. Dr. Morrison seems to stand squarely between the two groups. At the time he wrote his book he was espousing a low-fat diet, but he also used lecithin along with vitamins and minerals. He, too, by this method reversed atherosclerosis, painful angina, and other circulatory ailments.

Since you have already seen what the Longevity Institute has accomplished with its method (the low-fat diet plus exercise), let me give you two examples of recovery reported by Richard A. Passwater, an advocate of the second school of thought.

Jacobus Rinse, Ph.D., at the age of fifty-one, was found to have atherosclerosis as well as painful angina, complicated by heart spasms. He did not smoke, was not overweight, had no unusual tensions, and took sufficient exercise. He had no family history of this disease. Completely baffled, he decided he must have some nutritional deficiency, and after reading the literature avidly, decided to add one tablespoon of lecithin granules to his breakfast cereal.

He noticed good results within a few days. The heart spasms ceased, and by the end of three months all signs of angina, even after exercising, had stopped. A year later he could again resume outdoor work and running. Even though he still could not believe it, there was no recurrence of angina up to sixteen years later, at which time he made the report.

In a group of Europeans, observed by a European physician, heart attacks in one and a blood clot in another also responded to lecithin therapy. In the second case, a strict diet without eggs or butter was first used, with no improvement. Still another man, at seventy-two, who had suffered several heart attacks as well as angina, stated that he cured himself with the lecithin therapy *in three months.*

In the above cases the lecithin was included in a breakfast mixture, originated by Dr. Rinse, containing brewers yeast, wheat germ, bone meal, one table-spoon of vegetable oil, as well as the tablespoon of lecithin granules (doubled in severe cases of atherosclerosis). These ingredients could also be taken in other ways, such as in a protein drink. In addition to the foods mentioned, supplements including 500 mg. of vitamin C, 100 I.U. vitamin E, and one multiple vitamin/mineral tablet were also included by the doctor for his own program. His breakfast mixture is now available at health stores, or you can make your own.

As for the calcium deposits that the fat-cholesterol plaques seem to attract to the arteries or that may pile up in the joints of arthritics, the late Dr. Jarvis of *Vermont Folk Medicine* fame may have provided a solution. He learned that because calcium needs acid to dissolve and remain in solution instead of forming hard deposits in unwanted places, apple cider vinegar could accomplish this feat. He demonstrated it in autopsies performed after death on aged cows. Those whose rations had been "spiked" with apple cider vinegar showed reversal of joint stiffness. For human beings Dr. Jarvis recommended apple cider vinegar added to drinking water to suit their own taste and sipped throughout the day or at meals like wine. It is a refreshing drink, and many people report feeling better after adopting this practice. Some people add a bit of honey for taste.

There are other degenerative diseases, resulting from other causes. Arthritis may be caused by an inadequate diet, as well as by too little acid. But it can also be produced by stress, a cause of many ailments. Stress creates tension, jams body works, slows down circulation, and prevents nutrients from reaching various parts of the body. All manner of degenerative ailments have been traced to stress. You will find a solution for this problem in the chapter on breathing.

One example of a stress-caused instance of arthritis was the man whose wife ran away with another man; her husband became a wheelchair invalid the next day. Meanwhile, if a heart attack or stroke should occur, it is no longer a do-it-yourself project. Call a doctor immediately!

There are other degenerative diseases which, due to lack of space, I cannot cover here, particularly since I have already written an entire book about them, including, among many others, such problems as high blood pressure and allergies. This book, *A Handbook of Natural Remedies for Common Ailments*, is available through your book or health store. However, the following pages will show you how to build health and resist illness in general.

### REFERENCES
(See *Bibliography* for fuller details)

1. Jon. N. Leonard, J. L. Hofer, N. Pritikin, *Live Longer Now.*
2. Richard A. Passwater, *Supernutrition.*
   ———. *Supernutrition for Healthy Hearts*
3. Linda Clark, *Stay Young Longer.*
4. ———, *Know Your Nutrition.*
5. Lester M. Morrison, M.D., *The Low-Fat Way to Health and Longer Life.*
6. Linda Clark, *Secrets of Health and Beauty.*

# 7

## Enzymes for Health and Youth

ENZYMES ARE catalysts that exist in every cell of your body. They speed up or direct the activity of various body processes. They consist of proteins and are highly specific in their functions. Enzymes act as housecleaners, and because of their many functions in helping maintain health, they are also called metabolic enzymes. We have much more to learn about these fabulous enzymes; the exact mechanism by which they act is not fully understood.

One category of enzymes that *has* been studied is the digestive enzymes, which help you digest your food. There is one type to digest fat, others to digest protein, and still others for carbohydrate and cellulose digestion. If you do not manufacture enough of your own digestive enzymes, you can buy them at a health store to help boost your own dwindling supply.

A nutritional doctor told me recently: "I would not be alive today if it were not for the digestive enzymes I take." The explanation is clear. You could have the best diet in the world, but if you do not digest or assimilate it, it cannot deliver the nutrition you need. There are some specific enzymes missing in some people for the digestion of certain foods. For example, many people throughout the world lack the enzyme that digests cow's milk. Cow's milk contains a form of milk sugar known as lact*ose*. The enzyme needed to digest lactose is lact*ase*. (Many enzymes have the *ase* ending.) Babies can suffer from this enzyme lack as well as adults. A health store owner recently told me: "I cannot drink cow's milk. I swell up with gas that lasts all day."

This person is not alone in such a reaction to cow's milk or anything made with it—yogurt, cheese of all kinds, etc. Many people know they are allergic to "something," not dreaming it is milk, which they may love. It is a common problem throughout the world. I am sympathetic, since I too am a milk intolerant. Whereas a few can tolerate soured milks such as yogurt or kefir, I cannot enjoy even these. This reaction to milk is not called an allergy but an *intolerance*.

Fortunately, a solution to this serious problem has appeared. A new product known as *Milk Digestant* has been formulated. It contains lactase, the enzyme lacking in milk intolerants. The product is in tablet form and is taken orally prior to any meal containing cow's milk. For those who have tried it (and I am one) it works like a charm. But it must be taken *before*, not *during* or *after*, a meal. This product, because the ingredients previously have been scarce, has been hard to find. Health stores are now stocking it as fast as possible, as it is becoming more readily available. I have been receiving letters from many who are delighted they can now drink milk again, thanks to this excellent enzyme product.

Because milk is used in cooking and in such foods as soups, sauces, and many others, I always carry my milk digestant tablets with me when I eat away from home, even at a friend's house, and take two for insurance before a meal. Beware of substitutes.

Some people who cannot tolerate cow's milk can use goat's milk. Others cannot. Fortunately, I can. I use goat's milk that I buy directly from a goat owner. Stores are not allowed to sell goat's milk in many states because of an ordinance requiring all milk to be pasteurized. If the animals are clean, tested regularly, and the milk, milkers, and containers are hygienically clean, bacteria count has been found to be lower in raw than in pasteurized milk. Also, raw milk contains enzymes. Pasteurized milk does not. Dr. Bernard Jensen states that the weakest and most sensitive stomachs thrive on goat's milk, and many people owe their health to it.[1] Most people do not need lactase to digest it.

Raw foods contain enzymes that can bolster your own metabolic enzymes. But these biological enzymes are destroyed at a temperature of 119° F., or to be on the safe side, above normal body temperature, that is, above 98.6° F. For example, if you cook a raw green tomato, the enzymes that could have turned it red are destroyed. So the more raw food you eat the better.

One doctor has claimed that if you are beginning to feel your age, it is because the enzymes in your body are becoming fewer and weaker. This results in a withering process, which is observable in people and animals. In fact, tests conducted on older people revealed that inadequate eating of enzymes in raw foods may lead to wrinkling of the skin, thinning of the hair, sagging of muscles and figure, as well as lack-lustre eyes.[2]

This does not mean that all foods need to be eaten raw. Some foods should be cooked, especially meat, which may contain parasites (such as trichina in pork). Also, some people, as they add years, are often unable to masticate their food properly. There are two solutions here. If you have no chewing problems, eat as many vegetables as possible raw, or undercook them as in the Oriental method of stir-fry, which leaves vegetables bright colored and crunchy, not pale and limp. If you do have chewing problems, get a juicer and juice your raw fruits and vegetables, which leaves the enzymes intact, or put them in a blender to make into soups. Freezing does not kill enzymes, merely inactivates them temporarily, but it does rob foods of some vitamins and minerals, due to the hot-water blanching process used prior to freezing. And the longer the frozen foods remain in the freezer, the greater the loss of nutrients.

But all foods need not be eaten raw. Some are even better eaten in cooked form. Carrots, for example, have been found to release more carotene (a form of vitamin A) than raw carrots. But if you do cook vegetables, don't drown them in water and then pour the liquid down the sink! Water leaches out vitamins and minerals, so cook them quickly in a minimum of water and save the liquid for soups or to add to vegetable juices. Another and very easy method is to steam vegetables. You will find a small, folding stainless steel steamer basket in hardware and department stores, which you can use in an ordinary pan with the water just up to the bottom of the steamer. Most vegetables take only minutes to be done, and there's no mess to clean up.

However, raw food enzymes are so important to health and appearance that some nutritionists advise eating at least 50 per cent of your food raw.

### Another Important Digestant

In addition to digestive enzymes, there is another important digestant, hydrochloric acid (abbreviated as HCL), which you can buy at health stores. It digests protein, calcium, and iron. Doctors formerly believed that HCL manufactured in the body begins to dwindle only as one ages. This is no longer necessarily true. Due to stress, lack of B vitamins, and other unknown factors, many people of all ages are becoming afflicted with this deficiency. Even some babies who do not thrive after birth have picked up and improved when given a tiny amount of HCL in their formula.

Although I have thoroughly covered the subject elsewhere,[3] I will repeat the highlights here. Many people, influenced by TV commercials trying to sell antacids, believe they have "acid stomach." Not only is this usually untrue, but even doctors who do not understand the widespread deficiency of this digestant may erroneously prescribe an antacid when they should prescribe HCL. The reason: *The symptoms of too much acid are identical with those of too little acid.* Although there are a few tests for HCL deficiency, including the unpleasant one of stomach pumping, you can find out for yourself if you need it.

Dr. Hugh Tuckey, now retired, is one of the few doctors who has thoroughly studied HCL and has done years of research on the subject. After trying many different compounds of HCL, he has found that *Hydrochloric Acid, Betaine, with Pepsin* (available at health stores) is the most effective and easiest to take. To determine whether you need it, or if so, how much, Dr. Tuckey suggests taking one tablet after your main protein meal. If you experience any uncomfortable symptoms, such as burning, he suggests drinking a full glass of water immediately to wash it away. At the next protein meal, try only a half tablet, he says. Gradually you learn how much suits your needs and at which meal to take it.

People vary in the need for HCL, even on a daily basis. Extreme fatigue or stress at mealtime stops its manufacture, so watch it! Think or discuss only pleasant subjects while eating. Incidentally, I know several people who manufacture no HCL at all. Two of them were born with this deficiency; the other acquired a partial loss along the way. I have received letters from numerous readers who told me that their gas and other digestive problems disappeared upon taking HCL. So not only does the need vary in different people, but many people who should be taking protein and are not doing so believe that protein does not agree with them. They are so right! They lack this compound needed to digest the protein.

The digestive enzyme that helps the body to handle starch, or carbohydrates, is called *amylase*. Still more important is a digestive enzyme that digests fat! This is called *lipase,* and could it be an overlooked factor in those with artery clogging? It is possible that the fats, instead of being digested, are being deposited in the arteries instead of dissolved and mobilized out of the body. Lipase and other digestive enzymes described below are available at health stores. Read the labels on digestive enzyme containers to be sure they contain what you need.

Other enzymes include *trypsin* and *chymotrypsin,* derived from the pancreas, which help pancreas digestion. Some people who suffer from pancreatitis apparently cannot digest carbohydrates; others cannot digest fats. My own mother was one of the latter types. When her doctor discovered that she had a defective pancreas, he restricted her diet to a pitiful number of foods for the rest of her life. I supplied her with the whole pancreatin product (from a health store), which contains all the pancreatic enzymes, and she ate whatever she wanted from that time on for twenty-five years before she died of other causes.

You will have to learn to analyze what enzymes you may need. More people may have a fat intolerance than may be realized. Gas can result from fat intolerance, as well as from protein indigestion or from intolerance to cow's milk. Dr. Lester M. Morrison[4] tells of a woman patient who could tolerate no fat at all. If she ate any, she became so bloated she was often embarrassed by friends who congratulated her on her pregnancy.

Although the former method of preventing fat intolerance was to put people on a strict fat-free diet, the newer approach is to use perhaps a medium amount of fat to lighten the burden on the body and supply fat-digesting enzymes and vitamins. These include not only lipase, but vitamin B6, and, in some cases, *occasional* bile salts. Lecithin is also a tremendous help.

Health stores stock various kinds of digestive enzymes, some separately, others in combination, since it has been noted that if one digestive enzyme is at low ebb, others may be too.

Watch your carbohydrates! Man-made concoctions like pies, cakes, cookies, candies, sugary desserts, as well as alcohol, and too many cooked foods create a great drain on the digestive enzyme system. Natural foods, such as raw fruits and vegetables, contain their own enzymes. Fresh fruits are a better choice for those with a "sweet tooth" than man-made "dead food sweets." But do not overdo even fresh fruits. Nutritionists are learning that, because of their sugar content, even though natural, no more than two fruits eaten daily is preferable to going on an unlimited raw fruit binge.

To summarize why enzymes are so important, here are some statements from two researchers on the subject. Few chemists or biochemists really understand the full function of enzymes, so the following information from those who are experts on the subject is indeed valuable.

Dr. Justa Smith, a noted biochemist and former Director of Research, Department of Nutrition, Rosary Hill College, Buffalo, New York, says: "Body cells are largely controlled by enzymes."

Dr. Edward Howell, a scientist who has spent forty years in studying enzymes,[5] feels that enzymes may spell the difference between health and disease, even life or death. He also feels that too few enzymes cause premature aging. Since cooking at a temperature of 119° F., he says, destroys enzymes, the body, al-though it contains many enzymes for many different purposes, becomes eventually depleted because of eating so much cooked food. It puts a great burden on the body enzyme system, including defense against disease. Dr. Howell believes that by adding digestive enzymes to our meals to balance the cooked food we eat, and by adding raw food wherever possible, we relieve the body's burden of a limited enzyme potential. Since some people cannot tolerate a 100 per cent raw diet, Dr. Howell's solution is to compensate for the cooked food you do eat with enzymes from as much raw food as you can eat, plus digestive enzyme supplements (from health stores). If you dry your own foods, he cautions you to use a temperature no higher than 110° F. He also favors freeze drying. Dr. Howell believes that digestive enzymes should be taken *with* your meals, not at the end of the meal. Otherwise your body may have already started to deplete its own enzyme supply. He also believes that enzymes are a missing link in health and well-being, as well as a factor in premature aging.

Do not ask your health food operator to tell you what digestive enzyme product to use. Outside pressures leveled against health stores can claim they are "prescribing medicine without a license," and the operator could land in jail. (It has happened.) Ask to see all of the digestive enzymes in stock, read the labels, and decide for yourself. You may have to try several before eventually finding the one that suits you best.

### REFERENCES
(See *Bibliography* for fuller details)

1. Bernard Jensen, *World Keys to Health and Long Life.*
2. Linda Clark, *Stay Young Longer.*
3. ———, *Secrets of Health and Beauty.*
4. Lester M. Morrison, M.D., *The Low-Fat Way to Health and Longer Life.*
5. Edward Howell, M.D., "The Status of Food Enzymes in Digestion and Metabolism," *Chemical Abstracts and Biological Abstracts,* 1946 edition.

# 8

## Other Foods
## for Rejuvenation

DR. JOSÉ FROIMOVICH of Chile has proved that the correct nutrients can help rehabilitate the aging. Dr. Froimovich is not a Johnny-come-lately to this field. He has been a specialist in gerontology for over thirty-five years. He has been nominated for the Nobel Prize in Medicine for his successful work in reversing or postponing aging by a formula he developed known as FGF-60. It also maintains the body tissue, he says, of people in all age brackets.

Dr. Froimovich explains: "All studies show that people should live between 100 and 120 years. The fact that most people don't is that at one time or another their systems are deprived of certain substances."

Dr. Froimovich's formula, FGF-60, is a combination of sixty vitamins, minerals, hormones, and extracts of organs, all of which he considers necessary to retard aging. He says: "We can reverse many of the symptoms of aging, although we do not claim this to be rejuvenation. By using FGF-60 a person can see a little better, hear a little better, have a better love life, have more strength.''

The formula can apparently prevent such diseases associated with old age as stroke and heart attack. Wrinkles become smoother, hair stops falling, energy increases. People who begin the use of this formula can in many cases soon play strenuous sports with safety.

Dr. Froimovich has performed over 15,000 tests with a hundred men and fifty women. The patients were approximately seventy-five years old and were subjected to nearly every known medical test before and after the administration of the formula.

A film has been made showing the progress of the patients on FGF-60, which was supplied in capsules, some for men, others for women (presumably differing only in male and female sex hormones). The film shows the elderly patients entering Dr. Froimovich's clinic on canes, crutches, in wheelchairs, and on stretchers. Thirty days after treatment the same patients are shown taking exercises such as walking, running, jogging, even playing basketball. One before-and-after photograph (published in *The National Tattler,* August 4, 1975) shows a seventy-six-year-old man before taking the formula. He looks closer to ninety. In the picture, taken three years later when he was seventy-nine, he looks closer to forty.

Now I am sure you are all agog as to where you can purchase this formula. You can't, at least not in the United States. It is, of course, available in other countries. The FDA is holding up its release to the public here, although the substance is natural, apparently needed by the body, and has been found to cause no side effects or allergic reactions.

In the mid-1970's it was estimated that it would be three years before it would be available for sale. But those who have watched the FDA for many years are not so optimistic. It took the FDA forty years to release vitamin C to the American public after its discovery. And it took thirty years for the release of vitamin E in this country, although it had already been accepted in virtually every other major country in the world. Finally, due to pressure from both scientists and the public, the FDA reluctantly declared vitamin E essential for human nutrition. And then the amount recommended was so infinitesimal that few people got results.[1]

So don't hold your breath! When it is cleared, Formula FGF-60 will be available from Selfco, Inc., 8730 Wilshire Blvd., Suite 500, Beverly Hills, California 90211. I do not know the exact ingredients of Dr. Froimovich's formula, nor would I presume even to guess at the work of such a distinguished scientist. But as a nutrition researcher for many years I can suggest many of the probable essentials the body needs for repair, based on years of study by other scientists. I am sure that Dr. Froimovich, in the light of the FDA delay, would not hold it against us if we were to try to help ourselves with what nutritional information is now available. In fact, if we don't take advantage of such knowledge, some people may not be here when the formula is released!

Nutritional scientists have already isolated more than sixty nutrients the body needs for health, cell, and gland building. These nutrients include all known vitamins, minerals, hormones, glandular substances, as well as certain fats and special foods.

Since we do not yet have access to the Froimovich formula, and since there is no monopoly on nutritional knowledge already available, in self-defense we will have to look elsewhere for similar help. At this point I called in several nutritional consultants to help set up a program to bring similar results in the reversal of aging. You can begin to use this new program *now* without further delay. Who knows? This program may contain even more helpful information not found elsewhere, perhaps even in the Froimovich program. You will find it in this book, beginning with the next chapter.

REFERENCES
(See *Bibliography* for fuller details)

1. Linda Clark, *Know Your Nutrition*.

# 9

## Beginning Your
## Rejuvenation Program

THE INFORMATION in the following chapters is your passport to rejuvenation, providing it is used properly by adjusting it to your own individual needs.

We are all different. Roger J. Williams, Ph.D., a famous biochemist of the University of Texas, has written many books on this subject. He points out that each of us is as different as our fingerprints, our blood types, and in many other unsuspected ways, yet we can still be considered "normal." He calls attention to the fact that hearts, livers, and other organs pictured in medical textbooks vary in shape and size from person to person. No two are exactly alike.

Another example of individual difference: A recent newspaper article reported that one woman was found to have a heart on her *right* side, even though everyone knows it should be on the *left* side! Yet this woman is considered to be in "normal" health.

Textbook pictures of stomachs also vary. Is it any wonder then that digestion and assimilation may vary from person to person? Recent research proves that they do.

One of the first steps to take in your rejuvenation program is to start giving your body proper fuel to help wake up your glands, improve your cells, and increase your energy. There are certain foods that can act as tools to accomplish these goals. Some substances are basic needs for everyone. Others must be chosen for your own individual needs. For example, we all need water to drink. We all need food, and since so much food these days is refined or filled with additives and chemicals for coloring, preservation, and other reasons, vitamins and minerals have been pushed out to make room for the additives. So usually we also need vitamin and mineral supplements to replace those that have been removed from our food. The question is, What supplements do you need? How many? How strong (meaning what potency) should they be? This is where individual differences come into the picture. Vitamin A is a good example.

Some people need and can safely take huge amounts of vitamin A. Yet I, for one, cannot take any at all. So I have to choose *foods* that contain vitamin A in order to get my allotment. After all, to get well and stay well we really need *all* vitamins and minerals (which appear together in natural foods), not just one vitamin here and another mineral there. For best results we usually *need the whole works!* But since we are all different, one person, even members of the same family, may need more or less than others.

I cannot tell you exactly what you need or how much, because I do not know. To be absolutely truthful, neither does anyone else. The newer doctors are learning this fact, and they will suggest that you try certain supplements and see how you react to them. They believe that you know your own body better than anyone else, and since they cannot follow you around and watch your reactions from minute to minute, hour to hour, it is *your* job to find out what you need as well as how much or how little. We can all supply clues. For example, you will find each vitamin, mineral, and food described in my book *Know Your Nutrition,* showing what these supplements are supposed to do, have done for others, and *may* do for you. I cannot repeat the entire book in this one, so I suggest you look for it in paperback or hardcover at health stores to use as a reference.

Since you now realize that your glands and organs may differ from those of others, it will come as no surprise that you may not thrive on the diet that keeps your husband or wife or best friend in good health.

There are hundreds of variables between people. One person may be of a more lethargic, sluggish temperament and have a slower digestion-assimilation system. Often this type needs less food and does not get hungry for hours after eating. On the other hand, some people burn up energy rapidly, even in sedentary occupations, and a short while after eating they become ravenous again. These people may need more food, or may need to eat smaller meals more often, since their digestion may not be able to accommodate large meals at one time.

Researchers, including Drs. Roger J. Williams, Paul Eck, George Watson, the late Mary M. B. Allen, Arthur Robinson, who is a chemist and director of the

Linus Pauling Institute (all Ph.D.'s); as well as Dr. Edward Howell and William Donald Kelley, D.D.S., nutrition researcher, are turning up some surprising findings. It appears that not all people should be vegetarians, but some will feel better, stronger, and avoid anemia if they eat meat, preferably beef, at least about five times a week. Since, according to these researchers, there are people who cannot assimilate some of the individual amino acids (protein factors), this meat diet would actually make *them* ill. There are others whom vegetarianism can eventually make ill! (You will find such an example farther on in this chapter.) Some people can apparently get all the nourishment they need from vegetables, fruits, seeds, and nuts. Others, even vegetarians, feel more energetic on a lacto-ovo vegetarian diet, meaning they include dairy products and eggs in their diet. So it is never safe to generalize.

Professionals suggest they you alone can determine your own digestive-assimilation type, known to the scientists as metabolism, and there are many variations or subheads within well-defined metabolism categories. For instance, disliked foods, allergies, or food intolerances can interfere with the digestion-assimilation of some foods for some people. Even the area in which you live may be a factor (due to air pollution, noise, and other conditions beyond your control), as well as climate (too much heat or humidity, which may take away your appetite). It is generally known that emotions can affect your metabolism. If you live or work for someone you loathe, you are going to become tense, which can, in turn, affect your digestion and assimilation. The best way to find out your own hang-ups is to outline a type of diet for a month that allows for your own idiosyncracies, follow it faithfully, then evaluate it before continuing further. You may have found that your body chemistry has changed or that you can or cannot eat certain foods you used originally.

Allow time, also, to make a decision on vegetarianism. Almost everyone feels better, at first, on a vegetarian diet, since it is also a cleansing diet. But for some people, if prolonged, anemia, weakness, fatigue, and nerve involvement may develop, which can be serious if not caught in time.

Remember that *no two people are alike.*

It is not fair to your mate or your children to force your diet on them, or to expect their diet to agree with yours. Each person needs to take time out for a trial-and-error period to discover what is best for him or her.

There is one warning in connection with choosing the foods you think you need. Some people brag that their bodies tell them what they need. There is truth in the supposition that we should listen to our body language, but this body language really means that we should notice what happens after we eat certain foods, not necessarily follow overpowering cravings blindly.

There is a "wisdom of the body," but there are also false cravings. These include coffee, excessive use of salt, sweets, alcohol, and tobacco. They are unnatural cravings and should NOT be heeded. They are all habit forming and can throw off your entire body chemistry if you give in to them on an unlimited or a regular basis.

On the plus side, for example, some people crave

sour foods. This may well be a clue to a lack of digestive acid (HCL), which you really may need. Even those wild cravings of pregnant women may be important body language, and should be treated with respect. I knew a pregnant woman who woke up one winter night and had a violent craving for seafood. This might be translated into a need for minerals (richly present in seafood). So listen to what your body is trying to tell you, but pay no attention to the continuous coffee, sugar, alcohol, or tobacco route. Taking a bit of protein (nuts, cheese, or whatever you like) may satisfy your craving, which leads us right back to a nutrient that has long been considered a *must* for glands, as well as for anti-aging.

There is much speculation that those who are getting along in years may be suffering from a protein deficiency, and those who also lack energy may be short in protein. This makes a great deal of sense, since glands, which keep your body running efficiently, are made of protein. Even if your metabolic type seems to indicate that you are a nonmeat-eating candidate, it is still true that you may need protein in some other form. If you are averse to meat, perhaps you can at least eat dairy products. Protein powders abound in health stores, and brewers yeast, one of our finest foods, is a powerful protein substance, yet contains no animal protein.

It is possible that you may believe you cannot eat protein because it does not seem to agree with you. This is perhaps because you lack hydrochloric acid, which digests protein (as well as calcium and iron). This you can add as a dietary supplement, as explained previously. So if you choose the right type of protein for your metabolism and add the digestive enzymes to help assimilate the protein, you may find your energy returning by leaps and bounds. One of my daughters, the minute she feels fatigued or slightly weak, rushes to the kitchen, stirs up a tablespoon of brewers yeast powder or flakes in water, tomato juice, or hot consommé (the canned variety is delicious), and her energy is restored within a few minutes and lasts for hours, quite different from the effects of a cup of coffee, or some sugar, which provides energy for a few minutes, then leaves you feeling worse than before, leading to a yo-yo syndrome of wanting more and more.

One woman told me recently that her boss, whom she converted away from being a "coffeeholic" by giving him brewers yeast at coffee-break time, will suddenly look a bit wobbly and say to her, "I know what's wrong with me. Will you please fix me some brewers yeast?"

The weakness, common to people who are always looking for something to shore up their energy, is actually a condition called hypoglycemia, or low blood sugar. Tobacco, sweets, or alcohol do not give lasting help. Protein does. But protein can do much more:

The word "protein," coined by a Dutch chemist in 1839, means "of first importance."[1] Don Cordy, author of *The Protein Book* (see *Bibliography* for publisher), says that after water, fat, and bones are removed, what is left in the human body represents 95 per cent protein. But we use up protein rapidly in our daily activities and energy expenditure. Even stress can use up protein. This protein needs to be replaced on a regular basis; some nutritionists believe daily, others believe with each meal. Don Cordy states: "Authorities on nutrition estimate that about 70 per cent of our population suffers from protein malnutrition. Our diets in the United States are known to supply too high a percentage of refined starches and sugars and too little protein of high biological value."

Meanwhile, we cannot ignore facts. Those who are getting older, please pay particular attention to the following facts:

—Our muscles, which include our heart, liver, kidneys, even our eyes, are basically protein. Lack of protein can leave them weak and flabby.

—The liver, perhaps the most important organ in our bodies after the heart, needs adequate protein to function properly.

—A hormone, a chemical regulator, is a protein.

—The genes, which influence heredity, are proteins.

—The secretion of the thyroid gland is a protein.

—Insulin, manufactured by the pancreas, is a protein.

—Secretion of the pituitary gland, a master gland, is a protein.

—Antibodies, which defend us against infection, are proteins.

—Enzymes, which control digestion and a host of other functions, are proteins.

—Hemoglobin, the red coloring substance in the blood, is a protein.

—The body must have protein to repair a wound, a cut, or any other injury.

Even your appearance and good looks depend upon protein. Without enough protein the muscles in your face begin to droop, skin begins to wrinkle. Researchers have stated that the withering of old age may actually be due to lack of protein.

Adelle Davis put it more succinctly: "Since your body structure is largely protein, an undersupply can bring about age with depressing speed . . . Muscles lose tone, wrinkles appear, aging creeps in, and you, my dear, are going to pot"[2] (and she does not mean the kind you smoke).

Many people who are getting older complain of not feeling well. Lack of protein can play a part here too.

Protein deficiency has been found to cause the following:

> Anemia
> Kidney disease
> Liver disease
> Peptic ulcer
> Poor wound healing
> Lack of resistance to infection
> Irritability
> Fatigue
> Low blood pressure
> Wasting, weak, and flabby muscles
> Poor circulation
> Mental retardation in children
> Edema (water storage)
> Poor vision

Since we have examined different metabolism categories, we now know that some people can be vegetarians, others should not be. (I have covered the subject of vegetarianism in depth in another book.[3])

Meat, fish, eggs, and other dairy products contain all of the essential amino acids (protein factors). If one amino acid is missing, the rest are useless to your body. So complete protein is important, which explains why meat, fish, fowl, and dairy products are found to have the highest biological value, and therefore are classed as complete proteins. Nuts, vegetables, and fruits do not usually contain either enough protein or all of the eight essential amino acids your body needs simultaneously.

Let me give you just one example here. Mary Jane Hungerford, a respected nutritionist, tells the story of a nineteen-year-old boy who belonged to a religious sect that required its members to be vegetarians. He was required, also, to eat only raw food. As a result he had a complete nervous breakdown, followed by a second one; developed a serious skin rash; was skin-and-bones, as well as mentally confused. He lived largely on fruits and believed (mistakenly) that protein disagreed with him.[4]

Your glands need protein to keep you from falling apart. They also need vitamins and minerals for best performance. But one of the best things to feed glands is glands! There is proof. Radioactive tracers have found that when you feed liver to the body, it heads for the liver to give it a lift. Brain goes to brain, pancreas goes to pancreas, or, more surprising, if you mix all these glandular substances together, the body sorts them out and delivers them to the right places. How about that for efficiency?

So pamper your glands so that they will pamper you and help keep you feeling and looking younger. There are glandular substances now available in tablet form, and I will tell you about them in the next chapter.

## REFERENCES
(See *Bibliography* for fuller details)

1. Linda Clark, *Secrets of Health and Beauty.*
2. Adelle Davis, *Let's Eat Right to Keep Fit.*
3. Linda Clark, *The Best of Linda Clark* (an anthology).
   See chapter "Vegetarians Beware."
4. Mary Jane Hungerford, Ph.D., "Nutritional Factors in Common Behavior Problems," *Journal of Applied Nutrition*, Vol. 27, No. 4, Winter 1975.

# 10

## Rejuvenation
## Therapy

WE HAVE ALREADY emphasized the importance of glands. But why are they so important in aging?

Although in a few cases during aging some glands can become overactive, usually at this time of life the vital processes of the body tend to slow down, particularly glandular functions, enzyme production, and cell rebuilding. Assimilation may also become inefficient, resulting in retention of waste products, toxins, and body poisons. This, in turn, can lead to joint stiffness, weakened muscles, demineralization of the skeletal structure, a loss of balance, or incoordination, and a host of other disturbances. Some people develop outright degenerative diseases. (These ailments can, of course, appear at any age.) Many investigators believe that the basic cause of such disturbances may be due to toxins or deficiency of repair material in the body.

Tests show that many of these so-called "aging" symptoms have been reversed in various degrees by the simple use of an improved diet and the use of needed digestive enzymes, vitamins, minerals, proteins, glandular substances, and other repair materials the body originally contained but which are now dwindling. Fortunately, they can be replaced, and the body can use the replaced substances as repair materials to heal itself. The rate of recovery depends upon how deficient in cell-building nutrients a person may be, how long the condition has existed, and how serious it is, as well as the rapidity of the body uptake of these substances. The biological-nutritional concept is a simple, and almost incredible, concept (to some doctors), yet it actually works. It has happened again and again.

If these concentrated substances—which are foods, not medicine—are taken *regularly*, the body can also use them not only to repair itself but to prevent future illness and maintain health. It is already known that living cells have been kept alive for indefinite periods by the use of such nutrients. (Dr. Alexis Carrel's experiment with the heart, discussed in Chapter 3, is an example).

Raw nutrients are often more effective for body conversion into repair materials than those subjected to great heat through cooking. Glandular substances derived from raw organ meats have been known for years for their therapeutic effects. The American Indians, after killing a buffalo, always sought and consumed the raw liver first. Even though fire was available for cooking, they had learned that raw liver was more effective than cooked. Today much of our food is overcooked, overprocessed (removing many nutrients sensitive to heat), and some nutritionists believe this is one reason for the increasing rate of physical—and even mental—afflictions.

It is for this reason that the rejuvenation program presented here is based upon "raw" glandular concentrates, meaning they have been processed at only 37° C. (98.6° F.) and still retain enzymes and other heat-sensitive nutrients. You have read, earlier in this book, that radioactive tracers show how a glandular substance, when given the body, can make a beeline to the identical gland or glands in the body to begin its repair work.

But where can you find this gland therapy? There are several methods of gland therapy available today. Some doctors specialize in this approach (I do not have their names, so please do not write me for them). There are also "spas" or clinics that provide such therapy. But you can also do it yourself in your own home.

If you cannot find a doctor to help you with his expertise, do not lose hope. You might prefer to consider a spa. Let's look at those that provide what is called fresh cell therapy by injection. This method of treatment was introduced by the late Dr. Paul Niehans, of Switzerland, and is now available to the public in a number of European clinics. Patients eager for quick rejuvenation went to the Niehans clinic in Vevey, Switzerland, where fresh cells, or glands, taken from slaughtered animals were rushed, while still warm, to the waiting patients and administered by injection. It is said that among those who were "rejuvenated" by the Niehans fresh cell therapy were personages of worldwide fame—the heads of state of various countries, as well as a renowned pope.

I have talked with people who traveled to Europe for this therapy while Dr. Niehans was alive. I asked them frankly if they felt it helped them. I received the same answer from an average man who had feared getting old and from an internationally known actress who makes no secret of her perpetual search for youth. I have since talked with a large number of people who have received similar treatment at an existing spa not located in Europe. They all report almost identical results. In most cases the effect was good, perhaps even dramatic, at the outset (for several months in some cases). But these good effects did not seem to endure for long, they told me.

Since the cost of the original Niehans treatment was so high, including travel, housing, hospitalization, as well as the treatment itself, which was extremely expensive, only the independently wealthy could afford to go once, let alone return for "recharges."

Nutritionists and other experts, who have studied glandular therapy from a nutritional standpoint, believe that an initial injection of fresh cells is somewhat similar to a quick recharge of your car battery on a frosty morning. It will restore your battery temporarily and get you where you want to go for the time being, but is also a reminder that a new battery may eventually be needed.

According to these experts there is a better way. If the nutrients (oral glandular substances, vitamins, minerals, proteins) are *fed on a continuous basis,* a deficiency will most likely not take place, or once the body glands have been reactivated, *the recharging will be continuous,* since they will be receiving the necessary fuel *regularly,* not on a temporary recharge basis only. Your body battery would regenerate itself.

It is no doubt true that if you can take advantage of

the injection method, the sluggish glands may be initially reactivated more quickly. Or, if you have the services of a doctor who can determine through medical tests exactly what dietary glands and other supplements you need, results may also be more rapid. In any case it is up to you to provide your body with the continuous or follow-up daily fuel needed for the cells, glands, and organs to perpetuate their health. If you use the do-it-yourself method, it may take a little longer to nudge your sluggish glands into activity, but not only can it be done, it *has been done.* So if you do not have outside help, you need not feel that life has passed you by. Even if you can take advantage of the faster injection therapy at a spa, it is advisable to follow it up with the continuous method through diet after you arrive home. It is also more convenient and less expensive.

There have long been oral glandular substances available from the Standard Process Company (see Product List for address) formulated by the late Dr. Royal Lee, a nutritional expert. The substances are called *Protomorphogens*, available in tablet form, and can be procured only through doctors, though of any type (M.D., N.D., D.C., D.O., D.D.S.). This is not very convenient for the average person, since a doctor may not always understand glandular therapy and may refuse to order them for you.

There are now available some newer gland concentrates, which are not *extracts* of glands but the *concentrates* of the whole gland. These are made without sugar, starch, salt, and for those who may be intolerant to some foods, they also do not contain wheat, corn, soy, or yeast derivatives. These products are processed at body temperature (37° C. or 98.6° F.) and are made by the Nutri-Dyn Corporation. They are available at health stores under the brand name *Search*. No prescription is required. (If your health store should not have these products under the name of Search, you can obtain the same thing by asking for the Nutri-Dyn cellular concentrate, or concentrates, that you feel you need.)

In order to learn which ones you need, you can order the complete list from the company[1] or ask for a list at your health store. If you do not have a doctor knowledgeable in such matters, you use the homeopathic approach for yourself, which is based on the principle that "like helps like." In other words, if you believe that you are having trouble with a certain gland, you can take the equivalent glandular concentrate for a while and see if it helps (it will not hurt you if you do not need it).

Caroline Cropp, nutrition consultant for Nutri-Dyn, has reported that many people who have used these products for one to six months realize suddenly that they are feeling better. Because good reports are coming in from their use, as well as because of the convenience of getting them in health stores, I have built the rejuvenation program around these glandular concentrates.

After you use the individual glandular substances you think you may need, there is a combination product that includes ten glands for maintenance and further preventive purposes.

But before you begin your home program and choose your glandular products, there is a preliminary step to take.

## CLEANSING PROGRAM

Because waste products may have accumulated in your body over the years, before you begin your rejuvenation program, you may first wish to give your body some internal cleansing. Waste products can clog the intestinal walls and other areas, interfering with the absorption of the new and natural repair materials you plan to feed your body later. Those who have first used a cleansing method report better and quicker results.

There are several cleansing methods from which to choose. You may already have a favorite one you have used before with success. If so, this may be the time to use it again. If you do not have your own, I will share with you the one I use. It helps me and has helped others. You may or may not find equal success with it, but at least it is safe to try.

I do not believe in fasting with water alone except under medical supervision. The reason is that though fasting has been recommended in the Bible, conditions in our times are different than in biblical days. We have accumulated and absorbed many contaminants and poisons from our polluted atmosphere, water, and food, which are then stored in our fatty tissues. DDT is one example. On a water fast alone these poisons are released too quickly into the bloodstream and can become a source of self-poisoning. Some water-alone fasters have become dangerously ill. A juice fast or raw vegetable or fresh fruit fast would be considered safer.

The method I use was originated by Stanley A. Burroughs, who no longer lives in the United States. He calls his program the Master Cleanser. I have found that for me it cleanses my body of stored poisons, toxins, and mucus; helps clean the kidney and digestive systems; improves the bloodstream; removes some unwanted weight that has piled up in the wrong places; and in general increases my energy and feeling of well-being. I always feel and look years younger after following it for several days (you can stop any time you wish to do so). You can even cheat occasionally (as I do) if the program gets boring and you prefer a change in liquids. Here is the Burroughs method:

Combine the juice of 1/2 lemon with two tablespoons of a specific type of sweetening, and add to an 8-ounce glass of hot water. These sweeteners are a *must,* according to Mr. Burroughs, to balance the lemon and achieve desired results. The only sweeteners allowed are any kind of unsulphured molasses: Grandma's, Barbados, Louisiana, or blackstrap. Some people who have trouble with these, since they are slightly laxative (though usually a good thing in a cleansing program), use pure maple syrup with Mr. Burroughs's blessing. He does not condone honey for this program.

You are to drink this concoction, he says, from six to twelve times a day, whenever you feel hungry. Be sure to use a straw. Both lemon juice and molasses, if left on the teeth, can erode enamel. In any case, rinse your mouth with clear water after drinking, just to be sure. Take no other food during the full time of the diet.

Most people use the mixture about six times daily. If you are not eliminating properly, Mr. Burroughs suggests an herb laxative tea, available at health food stores.

Mr. Burroughs assures us there is no danger in this program; the only thing you can lose, he says, is mucus, waste, and disease. He reports that healthy tissue is not affected. But he does warn not to vary the amount of lemon juice per glass.

Now what do you do after you have decided to stop this program? Here are Mr. Burroughs's suggestions. Eat, as often as you are hungry, a soup made of fresh vegetables only or steamed brown rice. He believes that you should continue to drink liquids freely for two days after coming off the diet and take no meat, eggs, fish, breads, pastries, or solid food other than brown rice. On the third day he believes normal eating can be resumed. Coming off the program correctly is crucial!

One of the benefits of this cleansing plan is that the molasses, particularly blackstrap, is rich in minerals, as well as being a natural laxative. So you are really feeding the body as you cleanse it. Any cleansing method calling for little or no solid food is uncomfortable at first, since your stomach is shrinking and putting up a fight. The first two days are the hardest. Usually, by the third day you couldn't care less, particularly since you are feeling so much better. Mr. Burroughs says you can continue this plan for ten days, but I believe each of us has to decide for himself how long to keep on with it. There is no point in letting yourself become weak, and I am inclined to think that *great* weakness is a sign to *stop,* or if you continue after that, do so only under a doctor's supervision.

The nice part of this cleansing program is that you need not really suffer from hunger. Whenever you feel hunger pangs you can drink the mixture or cheat with something else, such as fresh juice (but no solids), although I sometimes grind up the lemon peel in the blender together with the juice and add it for bulk. The peel contains the vitamin C complex, known as bioflavonoids, so is beneficial. It also helps satisfy hunger pangs.

Here is another cleansing method:

Dr. John R. Christopher, a well-known herbalist, has written a helpful little booklet called *Rejuvenation through Elimination,* in which he gives helpful tips for detoxifying the body. He describes an herbal mixture that cleans out the fecal impaction in the lower intestines or lower bowel. This mixture is not considered habit forming, does not cause griping, and is not a medicine but a corrective food. It is called the "Lower Bowel Tonic." I have tried it and like it. You can get the booklet, as well as the herbal lower bowel tonic, from health stores or write direct to The Herb Shop, Box 352, Provo, Utah 84601.

Still another cleansing approach has been contributed by Caroline Cropp, nutrition consultant for the Nutri-Dyn Corporation, which provides the glandular concentrates I mentioned earlier. It is well known that the liver is the filter for body poisons. Thus raw liver on a gland-to-gland basis has been found essential to detoxify the liver as well as the rest of the body, by easing the burden of the toxin-filtering process by the hard-working liver. "The whole body can benefit," says Ms. Cropp, "if we keep the liver clean." Some of these benefits, she says, are a more glowing and blemish-free complexion, relief from constipation, renewed energy and stamina. Ms. Cropp reports that her own teen-age son experienced a remission of acne by taking eight raw liver concentrate tablets daily for two weeks. For a pre-cleansing program prior to the rejuvenation program she suggests taking thirty tablets of the raw liver product daily for approximately three weeks (together with a regular diet), followed thereafter by five to ten tablets daily for preventive purposes.

### Choosing Your Glandular Aids

Meanwhile, she repeats, when you begin taking your organ concentrates, you choose them by the "like-helps-like" principle of homeopathy. In other words, if you have a kidney problem, you choose the kidney concentrate. If you have a thyroid problem, you would choose the thyroid raw organ concentrate. And so on. After the one- to six-month period, during which time Ms. Cropp finds improvement has usually taken place, you might wish to switch from the individual organ concentrates to the multiple organ product (called Multitrophic).

(Please remember that neither health store operators, nor Ms. Cropp, nor I are authorized to prescribe which organ substance you need.)

Some of the possible benefits reported to Ms. Cropp by doctors experienced in glandular therapy are:

*Spleen and Thymus* glands act to help the body's immunization against virus and infections. These glandular substances are available in the glandular concentrates.

*Placenta* has recently been reported by the Russians as successful for reversing or preventing aging. Dr. Niehans used placenta injections to help improve memory, promote better energy, fight fatigue, and affect almost every gland, including the sex glands. It is used extensively in cell therapy and has often turned the tide from sickness to health. Placenta is rich in RNA and DNA factors, so necessary for cell rejuvenation. Placenta is also available in organ concentrate form. Many women are concerned about using the sex hormone products, since there has been so much publicity citing them as a cause of cancer. Here is the most recent concept.

There is a difference between *hormones* (such as estrogen) taken separately from the sexual glands, which merely stimulate, and the *whole gland* concentrate, which helps rebuild or supply the waning body gland. The concentrate of the whole ovary can be used by menopausal women who have stopped producing estrogen. The ovary glandular substance can thus help the body ovary produce its own natural estrogen, which in turn may help body rejuvenation. This product is called Gonadotrophic F (female), whereas orchic tissue, which has a similar rejuvenation effect on males, is called Gonadotrophic M (male). (The Search brand ovary is called Ovinol; orchic is called Orchinol.) Prostate glandular concentrate has often helped regulate an enlarged prostate.

Raw heart glandular concentrate is designed to give support to the heart. Other products include the organ concentrates of stomach, digestive enzymes, lymph, mammary, adrenal, pituitary, eye, bone, pancreas, thyroid, kidney, parotid gland, brain, and uterus. In fact, a product for almost anything that is wrong with you is now available in a glandular concentrate substance. If confused about glandular names, write to Ms. Cropp at Nutri-Dyn (address in References and Product List).

In addition to glandular and cell substances you will need proper fuel for your body in the form of vitamins and *particularly* minerals—recent research has pinpointed that minerals may be a common denominator in non-aging. These nutrients are found in carefully chosen foods.

Now that you are off junk food, there is no reason to buy it or store it in your cupboard or refrigerator to tempt you in a weak moment. Stock up instead on natural foods, including fruits, raw vegetables, proteins that agree with you. Before long you should begin to feel and see the good results of your program.

Certain foods are more powerful than others, somewhat like high octane fuel, for the continuous repair of your body, tissues, cells, organs, and glands. Let's next look at these foods and other helps.

REFERENCES

1. Nutri-Dyn Products Corp., 5705 Howard Street, Niles, Illinois 60078; Search Labs, same address. Caroline Cropp is located at the Florida office of the Nutri-Dyn Company. Address: Nutri-Dyn American Distributors, 2320 S.W. 60th Way, Hollywood, Florida 33023.

# 11

## Power Foods

WE CANNOT LIVE on supplements alone. It would take a huge tablet or capsule to include enough of these nutrient needs by the body. Many nutritionists and nutritional doctors believe it is better to get the nutrients already discovered (plus the unknowns as yet undiscovered, which do occur in nature) in *foods* if possible, and then supplement the foods with extra vitamins and minerals in tablet or capsule form as needed. There are certain special foods, often called wonder foods, that contain more of the above nutrients than ordinary foods and thus help build stronger cells and provide more energy. We will look at these power foods shortly. They are a plus value and save you money, as well as preventing you from eating too many calories.

### Live Foods

Live foods, which are uncooked foods, contain more nutrients, as a rule, than cooked or processed foods. Live foods, as we have found, also contain enzymes of many kinds that cooked foods do not.

In addition to raw, or live, foods there are also lifegiving foods, something quite different from just raw foods. Brown Landone once wrote about such foods—he called them "auxin foods"[1]—which seem to carry an electrical charge or growth factor. Studies made on old, decrepit rats, the equivalent of ninety-year-old humans, showed that when given these auxins, or life-promoting, foods the aged rats were eventually transformed, and their bodies began to grow younger. One of the auxin foods is seed sprouts, like those eaten by the Chinese. Dr. Howell states that *sprouts have the highest concentration of enzymes of all foods.* They are also rich in vitamins as well as auxins. They are becoming available in many food markets, but if they are not available in your area, you can make your own.

There are many good gadgets on the market for sprouting seeds, but you can use what you have on hand: a colander and white paper towels. The seeds should be bought from a health food store, not a nursery, where fungicide or other poisons may have been used for coating them.

Choose from alfalfa seeds, soy beans, Chinese mung beans, or wheat or rye seeds. Soak a few overnight in cool water and in the morning rinse and place. on a layer of paper towel in the colander. Cover with another towel. Put the whole thing under the faucet and soak everything. Let drain, then put aside in a corner of your kitchen counter. Repeat the soaking process each morning until the sprouts appear and are long enough. Except for alfalfa and mung beans, they should be about the length of the seed itself. This applies especially to wheat and rye, for the longer sprouts from these become too stringy to eat. Alfalfa and mung sprouts may be as long as you wish.

When the sprouts are ready, remove them to a plastic bag and refrigerate. They will keep about a week. Meanwhile start a new batch. DO NOT COOK THEM or you will destroy the auxins or rejuvenating substances. Use in salads, or in place of lettuce in sandwiches. Eat some daily as snacks or add at the last minute to soups and omelets—to warm only, not cook.

Another life-promoting food is the uncooked yolk of a fertile egg. A fertile egg hatches; an infertile egg does not. The raw fertile egg is the food from which the small chicken grows, yolk *and* white, and to which it owes its growth and existence. Some people insist that the white is useless. Some day we will find that again Nature knows best and put the white in the egg for a purpose. If you read that fertile eggs are no better for you than infertile eggs, remember that most large chicken-raising companies do not have fertile eggs to sell. A fertile egg requires the presence of a rooster for hens who scratch and feed on the ground. Most chicken-raisers keep their chickens in wire cages. The hens never see the ground—or a rooster. To show you how important fertile eggs are, the heart muscle kept alive by Dr. Alexis Carrel for so many years was fed nutrients that contained incubated eggs.[2]

### Protein

You have already read that protein is urgently needed in order to keep your body muscles firm and your body machinery working properly. If you have a protein digestion problem, you also know by now how to solve that problem. Check to see if you need HCL.

## Brewers Yeast

Brewers yeast, sometimes called nutritional yeast, since it is no longer restricted to by-products of brewing but developed especially as a food, is one of our power foods. It contains most of the important B vitamins, all of the essential amino acids or protein factors (thus is a complete protein food), as well as the major minerals.

It is one of the greatest sources of energy available. People who take it feel a pick-up within about ten minutes, and it lasts several hours. It can be taken in water, juice, or broth. Most people begin gradually with one teaspoon per day and work up to a tablespoon. If gas develops, remember it is a high protein food (although it contains no animal products), and HCL can come to the rescue. It is even more powerful when taken with desiccated liver tablets. It comes in flakes or powder, is available at health stores, and because it contains so many nutrients is a bargain. The newer yeasts are far more palatable than the earlier varieties.

## A New Source of Oxygen

A new, exciting yeast has recently been imported from Germany and just become available in the U.S. It is called *Zell Oxygen* (meaning cell oxygen). It is a liquid yeast containing billions of live yeast cells and enzymes, is formulated to deliver oxygen to tissues and organs, and is being used with success throughout Europe. According to German researchers, this yeast product stimulates the bioelectric potential as well as metabolism in the body.

This yeast is not the same as raw baker's yeast (which reportedly can steal B vitamins from the body via the intestines). In fact, according to researchers, these live yeast cells (not killed by heat) do not reproduce in the intestines, yet they do help restore damaged intestinal flora in a comparatively short time. The yeast is cultured at 86° F. (30° C.), substantially below body temperature. The culturing process is somewhat similar to the culture of live acidophilus. There are 5,000,000 living, nutritional yeast cells per 1/5th teaspoon.

Zell Oxygen differs from dry, regular brewers yeast in that this liquid yeast contains live cells and enzymes, whereas dried brewers yeast is inert from exposure to heat treatment. Zell Oxygen yeast is a form of primary yeast known as *Saccharomyces cerevisiae,* an excellent primary-source strain.

According to the German researchers, Zell Oxygen yeast contains B vitamins, minerals, and amino acids (also found in brewers yeast), but the live elements in the yeast have been found to improve food assimilation, help regulate blood fats as well as digestion of fats, promote brain and nerve and liver function, improve circulation and help detoxify contaminants in the body from the many pollutants we are exposed to today. The liquid yeast, since it activates metabolism, is further enhanced by adding a B-vitamin complex product (as in tablets) to the diet, as well as coupling its use with exercise and deep breathing to encourage the increase of body oxygen to the highest possible level.

These statements about Zell Oxygen are not claims made by me or the U.S. distributors of this product, but are the research findings translated from the German scientific literature on the subject. These scientists have learned that as a result of taking this active yeast animals had a longer life span, a healthier nervous system, softer fur or more elastic skin, and exhibited higher levels of RNA-DNA in their tissues. Similarly, humans were found to develop a smooth juvenile skin, experience body strengthening and a feeling of well-being, with greater ability to concentrate and also both to fall asleep more easily and sleep the night through.

Here are some statements by European patients who have used Zell Oxygen:

One woman wrote: "I began taking Zell Oxygen after a serious operation that caused much loss of weight. I have regained the weight and have continued taking Zell Oxygen for four and a half years. In spite of my eighty-two years, I feel very well and am doing my own housework."

Another woman reported that she has been taking Zell Oxygen with buttermilk every morning for three years. (Some people take it with juice, others in plain water.) She says: "I feel so young and vital that ten months ago I started doing housework for my son's four-member household, a task that lasts from 7:00 A.M. to 8:00 P.M. All my friends are enthusiastic about my appearance and performance. Though I am seventy-three years old, they tell me I look like a young woman."

A man who suffered severe shortness of breath on climbing stairs reported: "After taking three bottles of Zell Oxygen, I feel reborn."

Zell Oxygen, largely because it is imported, is not cheap, but physicians in Europe believe that five bottles a year are sufficient to produce the therapeutic results desired. (See Product List for source in the U.S.)

### Yogurt and Acidophilus

Yogurt and/or acidophilus can keep your intestines in order. Healthy intestines have what is called benign intestinal flora. These help you to manufacture certain B vitamins and discourage infections in the intestines. Unfortunately, antibiotics kill the intestinal flora, and indigestion may result. Yogurt, or acidophilus, which is stronger, helps to restore and maintain normal intestinal flora.

Yogurt has been credited with youth-giving qualities. It has been used constantly by inhabitants of Eastern Europe, noted for their longevity and excellent health. It has also been found to be a *natural* antibiotic, and it has recently been shown that it lowers excess cholesterol. Vanderbilt University has discovered that the Masai tribesmen, partly because of their high intake of yogurt, are virtually immune to heart disease.[3] Most people have to learn to like yogurt. Try to cultivate the taste for the natural, plain variety instead of that mixed with sugar, jams, and other unmentionables. (Sugar is a no-no in nutrition. Not only tooth decay and hypoglycemia but heart disease have resulted from its overuse.) If you cannot take yogurt because of milk intolerance, use one or more tablets of the product *Milk Digestant* (see Chapter 7) *before* eating yogurt.

## *Lecithin*

Now for some dramatic news! As people get older their immunity system can weaken, making them more susceptible to infection. Vitamin C helps to forestall infections, but there is help against the virus problem and other disturbances by the use of lecithin. This information, which is almost earthshaking, was originally reported several years ago by Lester M. Morrison, M.D.,[4] but nobody seemed to notice it.

As you have already read, Dr. Morrison was apparently one of the first doctors to recognize that lecithin could emulsify or dissolve fat, and as he explains it: "Apparently lecithin has the ability to increase the esterases in the human bloodstream. These esterases are enzymes that aid in the metabolizing of fat or cholesterol."

But Dr. Morrison goes much farther. He says that *lecithin also has the ability to increase the gamma globulin in the body.* (Gamma globulins attack various infections.) Dr. Morrison states: "In the bloodstream of patients who used lecithin as recommended we found evidence of increased immunity against virus infections." He points out that scientists have also reported that lecithin can produce immunity against pneumonia and prevent a variety of other diseases, including rheumatic carditis, liver diseases, anemia, kidney disorders, and certain skin diseases, including psoriasis.

Others have noted lecithin's good effect on the brain. Lecithin is high in phosphorus. There is a saying in Europe, "No phosphorus, no brains." In addition, lecithin can act as a natural tranquilizer, since a high concentration of lecithin is found to occur in a normal body, not only in the brain, but in the myelin sheath surrounding the nerves, thus producing a natural tranquilizing effect. It is also normally present in the heart, the bone marrow, the kidneys, liver, spinal cord, and blood, as well as in glands, especially the sex glands.

Since it has also been reported to be helpful in dissolving gallstones, lecithin indeed has remarkable value for health. When an element is so widespread in the body, it is continually needed to maintain its level. So adding it to the diet regularly is an important precaution.

Edward R. Hewitt, a lecithin researcher, says: "It must be well understood that lecithin is not a drug; it is a food. There is no danger in taking it. It simply furnishes some of the materials the body needs for growth and renewal of cells."[5]

Dr. Morrison concludes: "Lecithin is one of our most powerful weapons against disease." He found it took about three months to reverse many serious conditions due to its deficiency.

I have explained earlier what kinds of lecithin to take and how much. I take a tablespoon of the liquid in fruit juice before breakfast, followed by a hot drink to help dissolve it. Liquid lecithin looks and pours like honey. Since it is sticky and clings to any container or spoon, I reserve a small empty jar for this use only. In the morning I add a tablespoon or so of cold fruit juice to the jar, followed by an estimated tablespoon of the liquid lecithin (to bypass a measuring spoon), and gulp down the whole thing directly from the jar. In a few days the lecithin will start to cling to the inner walls of the jar. This residue can be wiped out with a dry paper towel, or soaked and washed with liquid detergent plus water, or removed by both methods. An even less messy way is to swig it straight out of the bottle. I suggested it to one fastidious friend, and she swears by it. I also add a heaping tablespoon of lecithin granules to my protein drink, which I have for lunch. This consists of a cup of juice (fruit or tomato) or yogurt, plus a heaping tablespoon each of brewers yeast (I use Red Star yeast only), plus a protein powder such as Malabar or High Energy Multi-Purpose Food, as well as lecithin granules and perhaps a dash of desiccated liver powder.

Alan H. Nittler, M.D., the nutritional physician, writes:[6] "The use of lecithin for flu is fantastic. Take 1 tablespoon of liquid lecithin or its equivalent, which totals sixty 200-mg. perles, or ten 1200-mg. capsules four times daily for six doses." This remedy alone has cured many cases of flu. *Warning*: Lecithin is high in phosphorus and can cause an acute calcium shortage if this high dosage is continued. (This often results in leg and other cramps.) If you need more than one series of six doses of lecithin for flu, be sure to add large quantities of calcium, such as calcium lactate, to offset the calcium loss. Dr. Nittler summarizes: "The lecithin routine can be used for any virus infection, such as measles, shingles, or chicken pox."

The fact that women often live longer than men mystifies everyone. Years ago I came across an explanation that startled me and that I put in my book *Stay Young Longer*. Apparently nobody noticed it except one man, who told me he had read and followed the advice. He has already outlived other men his age. To my knowledge he is still following the advice. Greatly abbreviated, it is this:

Semen apparently contains lipoids, or phospholipids—mainly lecithin—which appear also in the brain and nerves. Doctors who have studied the subject found that seminal discharges can cause withdrawal of lecithin and its components from the body, depriving the arteries as well as sex glands, brain, and nerves of these substances, "which are of utmost importance for its nutrition . . . in other words the organism needs more incoming energy than leaves the body." Therefore, lecithin must be put back in the body to compensate for the loss.

If lecithin is added to the male diet to replace its loss through semen discharge, there is apparently less danger of a deficiency developing. Since lecithin is found to exist in many other parts of the body as well as these crucial areas, perhaps by keeping it in the diet at all times to compensate for lecithin withdrawal via the semen, senility could be lessened, nerves fortified, and life lengthened. Every wife would do well to serve her husband lecithin, as well as vitamins A, E, and B daily to insure his health, youth, and longer life.

### High Energy Multi-Purpose Food

There are many good protein powders on the market. One of the newest is High Energy Multi-Purpose Food. I like it because it tastes good, contains enzymes for better assimilation, and is also a predigested complete protein. It contains many high-powered foods: soy flour, alfalfa, lecithin, wheat germ (which contains vitamin E and protein), rice polishings (contain B vitamins), kelp (minerals), food yeast, plus B-12, as well as ground raw seeds—alfalfa, pumpkin (rich in zinc for skin, hair, and prostate), sesame, sunflower (rich in minerals, vitamins, and protein), flax (for skin and constipation), and Chia (for energy). This powder contains no animal products, salt, sugar, or preservatives. (For source see Product List at the end of the book.)

## Onions and Garlic

Onions and garlic are considered beneficial foods. Garlic has been found to be a help in lowering high blood pressure,[7] as well as discouraging parasites in people and animals. European doctors have fed onions and garlic to horses to reverse obstructions from atherosclerosis in the legs.[2] Both onions and garlic contain sulfur, a blood cleanser. Garlic can be taken in perle form. A recent new Japanese product, *Kyolic* (pronounced Kee-oh-lick), available from health stores, is a garlic extract in liquid form that you can add to your own capsules (included) to take as needed. This product leaves no unpleasant after-breath odor.

Recent reports show that garlic can be a rejuvenator too. In an article in *New Woman* magazine (March–April, 1978) Rex Adams explains that garlic produces a tonic effect on all parts of the body: skin, muscles, tissues, nails, hair, organs, and bloodstream, even the hormone glands. Adams, also an author of a book on "miracle foods," believes that garlic invigorates as well as rejuvenates. He claims this can happen within a surprisingly short time, helping you to turn the clock back in the way you feel as well as in the way you look.

The garlic diet suggested by Rex Adams is simple: a

protein at every meal as well as garlic in some form. For breakfast, toast could be spread with garlic butter; at lunch and dinner chopped raw garlic can be added to vegetables or salad dressings. He says that if you don't like garlic or do not want to be socially unacceptable, you can use, instead of fresh, raw garlic, a garlic perle or capsule (from health stores) before each meal. It is said that eating a sprig or two of parsley after a meal containing garlic will destroy the odor, at least temporarily.

Adams reports that garlic increases circulation and oxygen, detoxifies the bloodstream, and, when used with leafy green vegetables, helps to release vitamins, minerals, and enzymes from other foods. He cites other benefits of garlic in his book *Miracle Medicine Foods* (published by Parker Publishing Company, West Nyack, N.Y.).

### Salt Free Diet

In addition to a fat-free diet, many orthodox doctors are recommending a salt-free diet. Nutritionists frown on this practice. The body needs *some* salt, or sodium, otherwise disturbing problems can result. For example, the body requires some salt to manufacture HCL. Again, it is a matter of how much and what kind of salt. The average salt cellar on your table contains pure, refined sodium chloride. A whole natural salt includes many minerals in trace amounts. Using small amounts of salt may suffice, but its presence is still crucial!

There are available a few salts that are whole salts, meaning that they contain traces of many minerals, not just sodium chloride alone. *These whole salts taste and look the same as sodium chloride,* but are preferable in normal amounts to sodium chloride, taken alone. I use this whole salt exclusively. There are several types available in health stores. The one I use is a whole sea salt imported from France or Belgium, and is called *Chico San* salt. There are, of course, other whole salts available at health stores.

Too little sodium in the diet can cause great fatigue. Remember the warnings of heat prostration for which doctors have actually prescribed salt? This deficiency can occur at other times in addition to heat exposure; many times great fatigue can be traced to a lack of sodium. Why? Doctors may have forgotten that salt is an important substance, which provides a base for producing electrolytes in the body. This, in turn, helps to generate body electricity, or energy. One nutritional physician tells his heart patients, whom he has first checked thoroughly, but who still may have intermittent feelings of weak pulse, to put some sea salt in a jar, add water, and sip whenever the weakness appears. This "revs" up the body electricity and increases the heart's energy, as well as that of the body as a whole. Patients report remarkable relief. (This should be done under medical supervision.)

Do not be hoodwinked by a label on any container stating that a salt is sea salt. It is probably from the sea originally, but, in the process of drying, the pure sodium chloride may be precipitated out and other important trace minerals that are so valuable eliminated. Therefore, it may be a sea salt, but not a *whole* sea salt.

**REFERENCES**
(See *Bibliography* for fuller details.)

1. Linda Clark, *Stay Young Longer.*
2. Richard A. Passwater, *Supernutrition for Healthy Hearts.*
3. *Natural Food and Farming*, Atlanta, Texas, February 1975, p. 48.
4. Lester M. Morrison, M.D., *The Low-Fat Way to Health and Longer Life.*
5. Linda Clark, *Secrets of Health and Beauty.*
6. Alan H. Nittler, M.D., *A New Breed of Doctor.*
7. Linda Clark, *Handbook of Natural Remedies for Common Ailments.*

# 12

## Other Helps for
## Rejuvenation

*Minerals*

WITHOUT MINERALS vitamins cannot work properly. Minerals are now considered by some even more important than vitamins. Both are necessary. Enzyme activity is also dependent on minerals.

Recent research by doctors and scientists indicates that minerals not only help to slow down aging; they help you live longer, feel better, and look younger. These same researchers have learned that a lack of minerals can cause fatigue, sleeplessness, poor skin and muscle tone, vision problems, joint stiffness, and premature aging.

John A. Myers, M.D., a mineral researcher of Baltimore, Maryland, calls attention to an article in *National Geographic Magazine* (January, 1973) by Alexander Leaf, M.D., Chief of Medical Services at Massachusetts General Hospital and Professor of Medicine at Harvard University Medical School, who studied the incredible longevity of the Hunzas in a mountain recess of Kashmir, as well as of inhabitants of certain areas of Ecuador and Russia. Dr. Leaf was convinced that the good health and longevity of these centenarians was due to a low-animal fat, low-cholesterol, low-calorie diet—*and* the liberal use of minerals in their agriculture and diet. Dr. Myers says: "It is my opinion that these people maintain their health and longevity from the activation of these mineral elements. . . ."[1] Dr. Myers has worked for years with minerals, and his word carries authority.

Mineral supplements, usually extracted from sea kelp, are available at health stores. A new product, called *Minerals 72* because 72 minerals are present in one product, is being used by an increasing number of doctors for their patients as well as themselves. (See Product List for more information.) Recent information suggests that minerals may be *the* primary anti-aging factor.

## *Vitamins*

Nutritionists believe you cannot eat enough of today's commercial foods to get the amount of vitamins and minerals your body needs to keep your cells in top condition. Although the FDA refuses to accept this statement, independent research has found it to be true. So you also need vitamin and mineral supplements. But you need not just one vitamin, you need ALL vitamins and minerals. In nature they do not occur singly but in combination. One helps another. Granville F. Knight, M.D., a nutrition-oriented allergist, says: "Since food is not what it used to be, we are all nutritional cripples, and need vitamins and minerals as supplements.'' In general you need the B vitamins for your nerves, your hair, your skin, and your heart. You need vitamin E to bring oxygen to your heart and other muscles; it is considered a youth vitamin. Raymond F. Bock, M.D., a practicing gynecologist, states:[2] "Vitamin E is the vitamin most deficient in the American diet.'' Dr. Bock agrees that vitamin E is a fertility vitamin. He uses it for menopause patients, heart problems, and fatigue. He says: "It increases muscular efficiency, combats muscular fatigue, improves general circulation, and therefore circulation to the muscles.'' He also finds that vitamin E helps alcoholics. He adds: "With an adequate intake of vitamin E everyone will feel better, look younger, and live longer.''

Dr. Knight claims that "Vitamin E is essential for the reproduction of human cells.'' Please study the section on vitamin E in my book *Know Your Nutrition* in order to learn what kind and how much to take. No two people need the same amount. Those who have had rheumatic fever or who have high blood pressure need to be cautious about taking too much. Otherwise you can feel your way, week by week, until you learn how much agrees with you.

Vitamin C is another oxygen carrier and helps you feel better as well as fight infection. Again, *Know Your Nutrition* gives you a safe guideline for its use. Please realize that I am not trying to sell books, I am trying to help *you*. If you were to buy all the health books available, they still would not cost you as much as one day in the hospital.

Furthermore, I cannot tell you individually how much of each vitamin or mineral to take. First, I do not know. As already pointed out in Chapter 9 in discussing what foods *you* should eat, everyone is different. What might help me or your Aunt Emma would not be the right dose for you. Second, not being a doctor, I would not presume to prescribe or even recommend dosages. I can *report* on what appears in the literature, and that is as far as I dare go. And for a very good reason. Recently I heard of a pregnant woman who visited a health store and asked the owner what he would suggest for her pregnancy. He specified calcium (which everyone already knows). He was jailed for his advice. The woman was a trap for a government agency, with a tape recorder in her pocket, and the health store owner was arrested for prescribing medicine without a medical license, even though calcium is a food and not a drug. This type of episode is not uncommon.

## How to Take Supplements

The best thing I can advise is to use trial and error in your own case. Your body belongs to you, and you have the legal right to do with it what you will. Always take supplements at mealtime, not on an empty stomach. Start with low dosages, let a week or more pass before increasing them. But be sure to read first what to expect. You can do this in my *Know Your Nutrition*, or in Richard A. Passwater's *Supernutrition*. Meanwhile, remember that you need everything, every day: raw foods, health-giving foods, all vitamins, all minerals, and plenty of protein, plus the digestive enzymes. This sounds like a big order, and it is. You really have to work at it, both by learning all you can about nutrition and then setting up your own program. It is quite different from the early youthful years when cells build themselves more or less automatically, yet can steal nutrients from the rest of the body when they do not get them in your diet.

If you want to be well, healthy, and active, adopting a program of good nutrition can be highly rewarding.

## *The Nucleic Acids: RNA–DNA*

There is recent research on RNA and DNA, abbreviations for ribonucleic acid and deoxyribonucleic acid, chemical terms few people can pronounce or understand. The point is that RNA is being commercially promoted for use in the diet as well as on the skin in creams for cosmetic purposes to help reverse aging. RNA is not something to play around with. If it is not used correctly (in oral doses), it can increase the body's uric acid, which nobody wants. Adding plenty of liquids and the B vitamin pantothenic acid helps somewhat, but I have talked with RNA research doctors, who prefer that you do not use this substance without medical supervision.

However, I have found for my own use, from many on the market, a type called *Biostrath*, imported from Europe, which is combined with several herbs. As each tablet contains approximately 50 mg. of RNA, though this is not stated on the label, it is presumably safe in this potency (see Product List).

Another product, called *Age Fighter*, containing both DNA (which involves the genes) and RNA (associated with cell renewal), has been formulated by Benjamin S. Frank, M.D., well known for his research on the aging process and how to slow it down. This product is available from The Prime of Life, Inc., P.O. Box 5107, F.D.R. Station, New York, N.Y. 10022. You can write there for further information about it.

### *Helping Your Memory*

Now for an exciting discovery for improving memory. A new product has become available and is causing excitement among those who are using it. It is an herbal extract made from a plant, a common ground cover, myrtle, or periwinkle (*Vinca major* and *Vinca minor*). Its value has been known since 1684. Recently a Frenchman, Dr. Paul Coupan, researched it with many patients who were suffering from senility, with excellent results. In drug form it is now available in Europe as *Vincamine*, which, according to this doctor, has halted, even reversed, the aging process in the brain, including dizziness, poor memory, bad temper, loss of concentration, and other symptoms of aging. Dr. Coupan, director of the Dausse Laboratories in Toulouse, France, states that *Vincamine* restores oxygen to the brain, loss of which is a prime cause of senility, and is said to halt the damage to the cells, therefore rejuvenating them.

Another French doctor, Louis Arbus, a neurologist at Pourpan Hospital in Toulouse, says: "The drug lives up to the claims that are made for it."

Still another, Dr. George Duche of the French Convalescent Establishment in Paris, reports: "We used *Vincamine* on 100 aged patients suffering from visual, hearing, and speech problems, dizziness, loss of memory, and mental disturbances. Nearly all benefited. It led to an improvement or total disappearance of the symptoms complained of.''

The drug *Vincamine* has not yet been cleared by the FDA for sale in the U.S., although it has been in use in Europe for some time. *But there is a natural, safe, and effective nondrug product available in the U.S., which is the periwinkle extract in natural form with no chemicals added.* It is taken in drops in water daily. People I know who use it report they can now remember names and other details they could not previously recall. One man could not even recall the names of people he had just met until he began taking periwinkle. Others who fell asleep in the midst of concerts or conversations (a common occurrence among older people) became alert once more.

Since this form of periwinkle is an herb, not a drug, it is well worth a try. It is not too expensive. Most people take five or more drops in approximately a half-ounce of water first thing in the morning. If they need more, they step it up gradually; some people need it twice daily, others don't. Taken at bedtime it can cause sleeplessness, since it encourages oxygen, thus wakefulness, to the brain at night, so taking it on an empty stomach in the morning may bring better results. (See the Product List for sources to which to write for information and price.)

## No-No's

There are various no-no's to avoid in your nutrition program. Sugar, refined foods, foods with additives, colorings, preservatives (read your labels) do your cells more harm than good. There is no point in eating junk food just to fill your stomach. Make every bite count!

On the other hand, don't feel guilty if you are invited out and your hostess serves you no-no foods. It isn't what you eat occasionally, but regularly, that counts. And when you go out, take your vitamin and mineral supplements and digestive enzymes along. It is getting to be the thing to do, so no one will laugh. More likely you will be envied your energy and good looks.

Surveys show that improved nutrition can prevent 300,000 fatal heart attacks and strokes each year as well as millions of cases of respiratory infections, 150,000 deaths from cancer annually, and substantial reductions in mental illness, allergies, alcoholism, arthritis, dental problems, diabetes, digestive disorders, eye ailments, kidney disease, muscular disorders, and overweight.[3]

Is it worth the effort to follow this new way of life? Indeed it is!

## Food Substitution Chart

| DON'T EAT | DO EAT |
| --- | --- |
| cooked foods exclusively | sprouts; natural, whole, raw foods |
| bleached, salted nuts | nuts in shell, raw or home-roasted whole nuts |
| chemical imitation flavor | pure extracts |
| preserved mayonnaise | natural mayonnaise |

| DON'T EAT (CONT'D) | DO EAT (CONT'D) |
|---|---|
| | (homemade or natural foods store) |
| Ketchup, A-1 sauce, etc. | homemade sauces, Tamari, soy sauce |
| saturated fats, lards, oils, Crisco, vegetable oils, margarine, salad dressings | unsaturated, unrefined oils (corn, sesame, sunflower, safflower, olive, soy, peanut); dressings made from these; pure butter |
| ice cream | fresh fruit-flavored yogurt |
| packaged, frozen, canned vegetables, fruits, soups | fresh fruits and vegetables in season; homemade soup; vegetable broth |
| Monosodium Glutamate (MSG) found in many canned and frozen foods, a commercial seasoning | dried herbs and herbal blends, kombu |
| dyed orange and processed cheeses | white raw cheese |
| baking powder, baking soda, preserved yeast | natural yeasts, living yogurt starters, unleavened products |
| chocolate, cocoa | carob and carob products |
| potato chips, corn chips with additives | natural corn munchies, rice cakes, nuts and seeds |
| commercial red meats (read labels for nitrate, nitrite, and avoid) | fish, fowl, organic eggs, organic beef |

| AVOID REGULAR USE OF | SUBSTITUTE |
|---|---|
| sugar and sugar substitutes (including saccharin) | fresh and dried fruits, honey, date sugar, molasses, maple syrup, sorghum |
| milk (pasteurized, homogenized) | soy and nut milks, raw milk, goat's milk, yogurt, kefir |
| table salt (sodium chloride), iodized salt | whole sea salt, sesame salt, powdered kelp, seaweed |
| tap water | tested spring, filtered water or mineral water |
| soda, coffee, tea | fruit juices, coffee substitutes, herbal teas |
| all commercial morning cereals | rolled oats, granola, oatmeal; whole, cracked, and flaked grain cereals |
| white bread | whole-grain breads |
| white rice | brown rice and other grains |
| commercial peanut butter and other bread spreads | natural peanut butter, sesame butter, and other nut butters |
| jams, jellies, preserves | natural fruit butters, honey |
| crackers made with saturated fats and/or bleached flour | whole-grain crackers; wheat, rye, rice cakes |
| candy, candy bars | dried fruit and nut bars; whole dried fruits |
| aspirin, antacids | herbal teas |

(REPRINTED WITH PERMISSION FROM THE BLUEGRASS ORGANIC CONSUMER ASSOCIATION)

## A Help for Nearly Every Need

If, after persistence in following the suggestions given to you to improve your health (which in turn helps to defeat aging), you still have some nagging symptoms that refuse to disappear, there is one more thing to fall back upon: homeopathy.

For those of you who do not already know about homeopathy, it is a system of reversing illness without drugs, practiced by some medical doctors who have elected to take training in its use following their graduation from medical school. Because it is safe, cheaper, simple, and competitive with drugs, it has been belittled, and there have been attempts to stamp it out entirely. The few doctors who still practice it have often achieved miracles where ordinary drugs and other treatments have failed. To find such a homeopathic doctor in your area, write to the National Center for Homeopathy, Suite 506, 6231 Leesburg Pike, Falls Church, Virginia 22044, for a free list of doctors who practice homeopathy.

Since one secret of homeopathy's success is to find the exact substance (often an herb or other natural substance) that is compatible with your symptoms, it will take a true homeopath quite awhile to question you and learn what your symptoms are. You will really receive full personal attention, not a brush-off. That the results are well worth it is attested to by thousands who have been taking these tiny sweet homeopathic pills, put dry on the tongue and swallowed without water. *And they are absolutely safe.*

However, if you do not have a homeopathic doctor in your area, there is a method of helping yourself with this amazing method. You will find all the information you need in an excellent book called *A Doctor's Guide to Helping Yourself with Homeopathic Remedies*, by James R. Stephenson, M.D. (It is published by Parker Publishing Company, West Nyack, N.Y., and is available on a short-term free trial examination. Just write and request that it be sent to you.) The book also lists the homeopathic pharmacies where you can purchase or order homeopathic substances by mail. I keep an almost complete supply on hand for every emergency. These remedies are far cheaper than most drugs and can be a real life- (or illness-) saver.

Just this week I was struggling with some stubborn symptoms that had defied all other treatment. Like many other people, I had saved the best for the last. Finally, I got around to this homeopathic book. I did some searching and studying for help for my stubborn symptoms, then took the appropriate remedies. In less than a week I was completely free of my ailments, though they had been bothering me for more than a year. (As I have said, I always learn the hard way. Had I turned to this method earlier, I could have recovered sooner.) Homeopathy has been known and used safely for hundreds of years.

REFERENCES
(See *Bibliography* for fuller details)

1. *Journal of Applied Nutrition*, Vol. 27, No. 1, Spring 1975, pp. 28–50.
2. Raymond F. Bock, M.D., *Vitamin E: Key to Youthful Longevity.*
3. Richard A. Passwater, *Supernutrition for Healthy Hearts.*

# 13

## Regular Exercise Can
## Rejuvenate You

WHENEVER THE subject of exercise is raised, most people start yawning—they think exercise is boring, takes too much effort, and requires self-discipline. These people would rather sit still and let others do it. Meanwhile, the others may go to the opposite extreme. They huff and puff and try to get back into condition all of a sudden. Some, when they find they haven't made themselves over within two weeks, give up entirely. Others continue to huff and puff, cheating at times, overdoing it at other times. Neither method brings results.

Dr. Herbert DeVries, Professor of Physical Education at the University of Southern California, says: "We've proved that any normal, healthy older person can rejuvenate himself to some extent through carefully planned and controlled exercise." The time spent is short, the rewards great. He states: "People ranging from 52 to 87, doing one-hour workouts in a leisurely manner *only three times a week* experienced the disappearance of long-standing migraines, headaches, backaches, relief of joint stiffness and muscle pain; reduction of nervous tension and body fat; lowered blood pressure; improvement of heart and blood vessel function, and increases in arm strength." There was also a 9.2 per cent increase in oxygen consumption after just six weeks.

Said Dr. DeVries: "The program was a real eye-opener in terms of increased vigor and sense of well-being in the elderly who took part." It is a well-known fact that high blood pressure (hypertension) can rise sharply, not only as a result of emotional tension, but with sudden physical exercise. However, if exercise is begun gradually and continued regularly, high blood pressure can be dramatically lowered by exercise alone.[1]

Exercise need not be dull, as I will show you shortly. It can be easy and fun. But why is it so helpful? There are several reasons.

As previously explained, diet is of primary importance in building the cells, thus helping you to acquire and maintain good health. But you also need exercise to stir up the circulation and distribute all those goodies you eat to the various parts of your body where the cells are. As people get older, they move less, and their circulation slows down. Hippocrates said, "What you do not use, you lose," and this applies to good circulation. It also explains the tottery gait, the stiffness, the cold hands and feet and other miseries of older age. The blood with its cargo of nutrients is just not getting there.

Another reason for exercise is that the lymph gland system, which contains body fluids to carry away waste, cannot move unless *you* move it. Exercise creates the necessary movement that carries away the body waste products, or "clinkers," from the cells, thus speeding up their repair.

And of course the increased oxygen intake brought about by exercise is a must for the brain, muscles, heart, and other functions necessary for good health. Have you ever noticed how former athletes who give up exercising often become some of the paunchiest Seniors in later life? I personally know one of them.

This man was at one time a world champion wrestler. He was not the usual Mr. America type with bulging muscles, but was handsome, well built, and lithe. As long as he was doing his thing athletically, he told me, his health was adequate in spite of a poor diet. But when he finally retired from the ring and gave up his regular exercise routine, his health went to pieces. He became a near-invalid. He was pain-ridden and looked fifteen years older than he was. Orthodox doctors, who tried drugs on him, said there was nothing they could do.

Fortunately, he learned about nutrition, improved his diet accordingly, and gradually rebuilt his health by diet alone, became handsome once more, and looked even younger than his age. The peculiar thing about this man is that with exercise alone, or diet alone, he was healthy. This should be a lesson for all of us. Why not build superhealth by using both?

A few researchers have already learned this lesson. The authors of the book *Live Longer Now* state: "Each of the degenerative diseases can be reduced in severity by proper exercise alone, although . . . *attention to the sort of food we eat is a prerequisite*" (emphasis added).

Now, if you have decided that you will, after all, get out of that chair and start to exercise, take it easy! Weekend exercisers only have not infrequently met their doom. After being sedentary all week and going on an exaggerated exercise binge weekends, they have done too much too soon, sometimes with fatal results. One doctor told me that on the last hole on the golf course some players could not resist finishing, and often died of heart attacks as a result. According to their co-players, they did not listen to their own fatigue warnings before they pushed themselves relentlessly "that last mile."

So whatever the vigorous exercise you choose, whether jogging, some sport, gymnastics, even yoga, for that matter, start gradually. If you were a tennis buff in your early years, you should know it's a pretty strenuous game. Wait until your doctor says you have built up your strength, vitality, and heart function before you tackle it.

What kind of exercise? I have some suggestions to offer, but recommend that you consider only something pleasurable to *you*. If you don't like bowling, for instance, you will merely tense up if you bowl. The idea behind exercise is to relax your muscles so that the circulation will flow, not be dammed up.

This applies to housewives too. They often claim they get enough exercise doing housework. Oh no they don't! I speak from experience. I hate housework, and it is anything but relaxing for me. There are a few women, though very few, who really seem to enjoy it. So unless polishing furniture and waxing floors is your idea of fun, cut the housework to the necessary mini- mum and instead walk, swim, garden, golf, or do anything else you enjoy. But don't clench your fists and tense your muscles and do your duty and kid yourself you're getting good exercise. It won't do you one iota of good.

Although I usually loathe exercise, one type I do like is using that pulley exerciser you hang on your doorknob. Lie on the floor, get all tangled up in the rope as it pulls your legs up, your arms down, and tightens your midriff. This I do with ease and joy. I started out with only a few movements daily and worked upward in number. The pulley exerciser is within the price range of just about everybody—it costs less than ten dollars. I have not met anyone who fulfilled the claims of making the body beautiful by this method, as the pictures promise, but the exercise is simple and easy, at least for me, and helps to keep you limbered up.

Jumping rope is a favorite of some people. *Live Longer Now* suggests roving. It means just that— sauntering leisurely through the woods or back roads, skipping or running now and then if and when you have the impulse to do so. You can also stop and rest when you feel like it. Above all, you can return home whenever you wish. Don't set any deadlines. Do what comes naturally. Only keep off the highways and as far away from them as possible. They carry too great a risk of picking up lead poisoning from car exhausts.

*Live Longer Now* also suggests bicycling. This is not for me, as I live on a steep hill. But another of its suggestions revolutionized my life. It stated that regular exercise, including bicycling, can decrease fat levels in the blood and that *a stationary bicycle is a good substitute for a moving bicycle.* So I bought an exercycle. It is the kind that works not only on your legs and lower part of your body by pedaling, but has handlebars and a seat that goes back and forth like rowing a boat, which exercises your upper body as well. I got it at a mail order house. I like it.

For those who suffer from high blood pressure there is further good news. Tests showed that regular exercise for seven months reduced the blood pressure of those who already had a high reading, and that exercise can help the condition at any stage.

What happens when you exercise regularly, experts explain, is that new blood-flow pathways are opened up, carrying fresh blood to the heart and other organs. With exercise gradually increased, the heart can develop more strength.

One warning: Whatever type of exercise you adopt on a regular basis, once you start, don't be wishy-washy about it. If you decide to take a day off, then two, then three, you have broken the habit, and it is hard to get with it again.

## *That Wonderful* Sundancer

Even though I like the exercise devices I have mentioned so far, I should amend this to say that they are comparatively easier than other types of exercises, which I really dislike. But to a total nonexerciser like me, even if I start and then get out of the daily habit, it takes willpower to get going again.

Not so with the *Sundancer*, which I tried first before learning of its benefits. It is not the same type of trampoline used by athletes, who do somersaults on it, but a small 38-inch portable circle on springs that stand about nine inches high. It stays set up at all times, without being noticed, so with no effort or willpower (it's fun) you can step out of your shoes onto the circular trampoline and bounce gently a little or a lot and step off feeling exhilarated, lighter, brighter, more relaxed, alert, and vital. At least that is how I feel after a few bounces. (It is not unlike bouncing on the back of a gentle horse while horseback riding.)

Here are some of the benefits reported by researches of this exerciser:

—Relieves tension
—Develops body poise, balance, and coordination
—Aids overweight problems
—Encourages circulation, especially of the lymph system
—Increases oxygen and lung capacity (as confirmed by tests)
—Stimulates vital organs, including the liver, pancreas, gall bladder, kidneys, and intestines
—Clears body blockages (especially in the lymph system)
—Increases energy, vitality, alertness
—Increases efficiency of the cardiovascular system (heart/arteries), as confirmed by laboratory tests
—Makes joints more limber

All this from merely bouncing, shoes off, feet flat on the *Sundancer*, as little or as long a time as you like. You can even pick your feet up and jog in a stationary position. Five minutes of jogging on the *Sundancer* are said to equal a mile of regular jogging on hard pavement or ground, now warned against for the elderly by an increasing number of experts.

The bottom of a *Sundancer* is so resilient that it can

accommodate a 300-pound person, and the mat on which you stand is made of Permotron, so tough that it is used in bullet-proof vests.

For those who feel somewhat unsteady or have balance problems, you can order a model with posts at either side to hang onto for security. A cassette for rhythm encouragement is also available. Or you can bounce to music if you wish. Or you can do it in peace and quiet, as I do.

This method of exercising is so easy you don't have to make yourself do it; you *want* to do it!

With such benefits so easily available, no wonder Dr. Corwin S. West considers it "a breakthrough in physical therapy," and other reporters state that "it keeps the fountain of youth bubbling." I believe it! (For further information about the *Sundancer* see Product List.)

Dr. David Kakiashvili, a Russian heart and gerontology (aging) specialist, states that exercise is a major influence in longevity. He has learned that people who live in small mountain villages have fewer heart attacks than those who live in cities. Their way of life necessitates constant physical activity, which improves heart function and supplies more oxygen to the body than is the case of city dwellers with their far less physically active lifestyle.

I have one other easy-does-it exercise to suggest. It brings oxygen to your muscles, which also include cells, and even if one is bedridden, it can be done by anyone, no matter at what age or stage of decrepitude. It also takes less than three minutes. (This leaves you with no alibi for not exercising.) I call this method Muscle Massage (MM). It is actually a tranquilizer.

I received a clue to this method when I read that Dr. Arthur Steinhaus, a former dean of physiology at George Williams College, had said: "In a German laboratory where I worked, it was discovered that a muscle can grow only at a certain rate, and a small amount of the right exercise will start it growing at that rate. If you contract any one of your muscles to about one third of its maximum power and hold it for six seconds a day, the muscle will grow as fast as it can grow."[2] This is admittedly an isometric exercise, considered by many ineffective. But good results are possible.

Where there are muscles, there are cells. Some of our muscles are voluntary, meaning we can move them; and others, on the inside of our bodies, are involuntary, meaning that we cannot control them at will. These would include our heart, glands, and some other organs. Even so, our bodies are really not compartmentalized. Each area nudges another, so that when we exercise the voluntary muscles, the involuntary muscles are also indirectly affected. So here's how you do it:

While you are lying in bed, in a bathtub, or sitting upright, you can tense and relax each area of your body.

—Begin with your toes. Squeeze them and bend them under, away from your body, and keep them clenched while you *slowly* count to six. This adds up to six seconds. (Say one hundred one, one hundred two, etc., up to one hundred six to slow down your counting.)

—Next bend your toes toward your body by bending your ankles. Your toes will not be clenched in this position. Hold for six slow counts.

—Now place your hands on top of your legs, between

ankles and knees. Tense these areas for six counts. Use your hands to help locate the areas to be tensed. They are temporary spot finders. Later you may not need them.

—Place your hands under your calves and repeat.

—Now place your hands on your knees and tense.

—You are ready for your thighs. Put your hands first on top for six slow counts, then underneath thighs, and tense accordingly.

—Next, tense your buttocks; count to six.

—The next area is a little harder. Sit up if you are lying down, reach behind you, place your palms on your back just above your waistline and on either side of your spine. This is the kidney and adrenal area (there are two of each), each set on either side of your spine. Try tensing or pushing those areas against your hands. Count to six as usual.

—Return to the front of your body for three more areas here. Contract your stomach muscles, then your rib cage, and then your chest (which houses your lungs, heart, thymus). Push each area against your hands, counting six slow times for each. Don't hurry.

—Your shoulders will take a bit of doing too. Put one hand on the opposite shoulder, hunch your shoulder, and tense. Repeat with the other one.

—Clench your hands, then the lower arms, then the upper arms. Count six for each.

—Place your hands on the front of your neck, then on the sides, and finally at the back of your neck, in each position tensing to six counts, then relaxing. Great tension can accumulate in the neck. (These neck tension positions help firm the neck and smooth away some of that flabby look.)

Since you need extra relaxation here, an additional exercise is invaluable at this point. Use the head roll exercise. Sit up straight, stretch your neck, and keep it that way. Now roll your head slowly in a complete circle, three times to the right, three times to the left. This also helps circulation reach the face, the eyes, ears, even the scalp.

—Clench your teeth and jaws. Count six.

—Put your hands on your cheeks and tense, then on your forehead, ditto.

—Now, *very important*, take your two index fingers and place lightly on each eye. Tense each eyeball. Repeat twice for the count of six, especially if your eyes are weak.

—Finally, spread your fingers apart, lay them on top of your head, bracing them with your thumbs placed behind your ears. Now pitterpatter your fingers all over the top of your head. You will be amazed at the circulation you detect in your head as you finish. This does not require counting.

—Most important of all, now do the all-over clench. Stand up, if possible, and slightly flex your knees and your elbows. Tense your entire body, holding for the same count of six.

The all-over clenching routine is absolutely safe. It was developed by two doctors to reduce high blood pressure. There were no side effects and nothing but good results noted in all people tested.[3] Blood pressure dropped when it was high.

If you don't believe this MM routine takes less than three minutes, time it! Do it once daily.

Since more vigorous exercise helps to reduce blood fat, add some other more active exercise of your choice. Watch out for indiscriminate jogging without your doctor's advice. Reports are accumulating that doing too much too soon can be dangerous. Again, let your heart become accustomed to exercise gradually. Never overexert at any stage.

## A Surprising Secret of Health

Recently a new secret of a cause of illness and pain made its appearance in our country. This may well shake up the whole world before long. Various world cultures have always believed that there is a vital force within our bodies. English-speaking scientists and others call it *Life Force*. The Hindus or Indian Yogis call it *Prana*. The Chinese call it *Chi*. Other peoples have other names for it.

This secret was revealed by Walter Delaney in his book *Ultra Psychonics* (published in 1975 by the Parker Publishing Company, West Nyack, New York). Mr. Delaney's theory is that *all illnesses and pain are the result of the interruption of the flow of the vital force in the body*.

This surprising and simple concept may explain the success of many therapies. Acupuncture needles are inserted at certain body points to release the congestion there and elsewhere in the body. Acupressure, which uses finger pressure instead of needles, has the same effect. If you do not believe this, investigate for yourself by pressing your fingers against the various spots of your body considered key points by acupuncturists and acupressurists. If you find a sore spot, it indicates, according to experts in the subject, that there is a congestion relating to some organ or gland in the body. *And it works.* Either by the insertion of needles or by pressure of the finger (the latter repeated daily for a short period) the soreness or congestion disappears, and the area to which the congested spot is linked responds likewise.This release of congested life force at various points could also be the explanation of reflexology, which is actually acupressure on the soles of the feet. It may also explain the success of Chiropractic and Osteopathy, through which certain nerve impingements are released, thus, in turn, restoring circulation of the interrupted flow of vital force in the body. No doubt osteopaths and chiropractors, and also some highly trained massage therapists, have always known this.

The relaxing method I call MM, described previously, can also remove interruption and congestion of the flow of the body's vital force. If you decide to try reflexology of the feet, you can follow the direction in any book on the subject and achieve results similar to those of acupressure. My favorite reflexologist is Anna Kaye, who has written a book with Don C. Matchan about it called *Mirror of the Body* (published by Strawberry Hill Press, 1977). Ask your bookstore for it.

## Non-Exercises

Once you form the habit of learning and using the MM plan, as well as the method of massaging sore spots in your body, you will no doubt feel more relaxed and normal. But if you want to try something still more unusual and equally effective—which helps rejuvenation as well as general health—you can use the system of *internal exercises*, another little-known exciting method of self-healing.

Dr. Stephen T. Chang, a Chinese physician living in California, together with Rick Miller, has written a book called *The Book of Internal Exercises* (Strawberry Hill Press, 1978). Dr. Chang believes that some strenuous exercises can be dangerous for some people, whereas internal exercises, which are more passive, are safe. They are designed to energize the whole body, balance the energy level, promote better functioning, and regulate the action of the internal organs, as well as liberate the flow of Chi (vital force).

In this book you will find through internal exercises some formulas for:
—reducing high blood pressure
—improving vision and hearing
—reducing the size of your stomach
—overcoming male impotence
—increasing energy
—reducing or removing wrinkles
and many more.

It would not be fair for me to give a full summary here of all the secrets in Dr. Chang's book. But he and his publisher have granted me permission to share with you three rejuvenating-type exercises. They appear in his book and have been known and practiced for more than six thousand years, yet are virtually unknown in the Western world. Dr. Chang states that anyone can become filled with energy, can become more youthful, and can begin to achieve freedom from disease through these exercises, which are natural and safe. Dr. Chang himself is approximately forty-four years old and looks more like twenty-four. His publisher-friend tells me that after a lecture, to which thousands of doctors have flocked, he may appear tired and somewhat older. But when allowed to retire to a quiet place for a few minutes, presumably to practice appropriate internal exercise, he appears young and fresh once more, the lines of his face lifted naturally.

Since this book is devoted to rejuvenation, I want to tell you about those of Dr. Chang's rejuvenation exercises based on the observation of three animals noted for their longevity: the deer, the crane, and the turtle. Here is a short, condensed version of each:

## The Deer

The deer, if you will watch it in action, waves its short tail back and forth constantly, which in turn activates and recharges, stimulates and strengthens the sexual and other glands. The human version of this exercise does the same for humans, and also strengthens the anus, prostate, and vagina, which may tend to become flabby in later years.

The deer exercise is simple, and you can do it anywhere without being noticed. Merely tighten the anal (rectal) muscles and pull upward as hard as you can and hold as long as possible. This exercise, according to Dr. Chang, can generate new energy all the way up to the head and to the glands located there. Although once a day is sufficient, first thing in the morning and just before going to bed are especially helpful times to practice this exercise. Or you can do it as you sit at your desk or table, walk across the room, or stop at a stoplight while driving.

### The Crane

The crane exercise, when practiced exactly as Dr. Chang's book outlines, is devised to help the abdominal area (including relieve constipation), as well as stimulate the lungs, circulatory system, aid indigestion, and promote a flow of oxygen.

For a shortcut here: Emulate the crane, which stands on one foot, folding its other leg into its belly. While you are doing this, first on one leg and then on the other (hold onto a chair or the wall if you need to maintain your balance), inhale and exhale deeply. There are illustrations and more helps in Dr. Chang's book.

### The Turtle

The turtle is well known for its longevity and performs only one major exercise—stretching its neck forward and pulling its chin inward toward the base of the neck, again and again. This exercise releases neck tension, as well as tension of the brain. It can also stretch the entire spine, energize the neck, strengthen the shoulder muscles, removing tiredness and soreness, and help to stimulate the thyroid, which, according to Dr. Chang, can increase energy and help you feel younger.

There is another type of exercise related to internal exercises that is more complex but very rewarding. It cannot be learned without a teacher, but is useful for everyone and can be started at any age. It is called T'ai Chi (pronounced Tye Chee), and to watch the slow, graceful movements of those who have learned how to do it is almost like watching ballet. The movements are slow, rhythmical, graceful, fluid, and beautiful. It appears to be effortless, can be done in ten minutes daily within a space of four feet, and without spending a cent once it is learned. The Chinese believe that if you do T'ai Chi twice a day regularly and correctly, in time you will develop "the pliability of a child, the health of a lumberjack, and the peace of mind of a sage" (quoted from Cheng Man-ch'ing and Robert W. Smith in *T'ai Chi*, published by Charles Tuttle Company, Rutland, Vermont).

So if an instructor in T'ai Chi comes to your area, by all means join the class!

Although T'ai Chi is newer to the Western world than Yoga and, once learned, is considered by many students easier to perform, the practice of Yoga may be more satisfactory and helpful to most people. The Yoga asanas, or postures, are not aimed at performing acrobatics, as many people seem to think, but are devised to relax certain centers in the body and aid the interrupted pranic flow. They require less training to learn than T'ai Chi, and inexpensive classes are more widely available in small communities as well as in large cities.

A recent, and excellent, book, *Yoga for People Over 50*, by Suza Norton (Devin-Adair, 1977), describes various cases of elderly people who have been substantially helped by Yoga, either self-taught or (which is preferable) with a few initial lessons from an instructor.

Suza Norton states in her book: "The American Medical Committee on Aging, after studying the subject for over ten years, did not find a single physical or mental condition that could be directly attributed to the passage of time. Such alleged diseases of aging as high blood pressure and arthritis are prevalent in the very young as well as the very old. *Many of the classic symptoms of old age are the result of little more than inactivity and inadequate nutrition"* (emphasis added).

According to findings reported in this book Yoga can accomplish many things for those in their later years. Its practice has improved or reversed:
—stiffness
—respiratory ailments, including emphysema
—high blood pressure
—lack of muscle strength
—accumulation of fat in the wrong places
—back pain
—heart problems
—prevention of senility in some cases
—arthritis
and other afflictions.

Now for a source of more oxygen and stress relief.

REFERENCES
(See *Bibliography* for fuller details.)

1. Jon N. Leonard, J. L. Hofer, N. Pritikin, *Live Longer Now.*
2. Linda Clark, *Stay Young Longer.*
3. Linda Clark, *Handbook of Natural Remedies for Common Ailments.* See chapter on High Blood Pressure.

# 14

## Breathing for Health

BREATHING SHOULD be automatic, and during sleep it usually is. But often during the daytime tense people unconsciously constrict their breathing or hold their breath, actually forgetting to breathe. You should check yourself at intervals. Lift your chest, drop your shoulders, then stretch the back of your neck (two common tension areas), and also check to see that you are breathing normally instead of holding yourself tense. If you are holding yourself tense, do some regular rhythmic breathing, choosing from any of the following methods. Breathing encourages more oxygen to the various parts of the body. It can also relieve tension or stress.

Captain N.P. Knowles, a breathing expert in England, says in the November, 1975, issue of *Here's Health*: "When you feel signs of aging, and wonder if there is anything you can do about it, there is one way: breathe."

Captain Knowles, who has rehabilitated many students through correct breathing, explains that as we get older there is a tendency to worry about trifles. This creates nerve tension, which, in turn, restricts the supply of oxygen. He has found that by daily practice of better breathing we can send a fresh supply of oxygen to the brain and ease the tension.

Here is the method:

"Sit in an easy chair and gently draw your shoulders slightly backward. Relax your arms and hands: then breathe out gently as if in a long sigh.

"Then, as though smelling a flower, gently breathe in, pausing a second to allow the breath to be converted into oxygen in the lungs, then slowly and gently breathe out again.

"Pause a second to allow the carbon dioxide in the blood to be exhaled. Repeat this breathing method 12 times and you will be surprised at how different you feel. Why? Because you have given Nature a chance to recharge your system."

If you do this simple exercise at the end of the day, Captain Knowles says, it will disperse fatigue.

The following method is used by Caryl Hill, who works with Seniors on the Monterey Peninsula in California. The Seniors are enthusiastic about the results. Here is the method she teaches these willing students:

*Step One.* Lie on the floor or a firm bed. Place one palm on your abdomen just below your navel. Place the other palm on your chest, close to the hollow of your neck.

*Step Two.* Take a deep breath through your nose. As you do this, your lower hand should (if you are breathing correctly) be pushed upward. Feel this breath roll upward through your lower and upper lungs to your other hand, which should go downward or inward or sideways.

*Step Three.* Exhale, slowly through your mouth, making any sound you wish—a groan, a hum, or whatever you feel like doing. This is a good way to relieve tension.

Caryl Hill explains that for best results there is a rhythm to follow in this exercise. Count 4 as you roll the breath upward, count 4 as you pause, exhale to the count of 4, then rest to the count of 4. (Later you may wish to work up gradually to the count of 8 for each step.)

Repeat the whole sequence seven times.

After learning how this feels while you are lying down, you can do the rhythmic breathing while standing, and then while walking. Some of the Seniors who live in a retirement center reported that they had had difficulty walking from their rooms to the dining hall. However, by using this method as they walked, they reached the dining room with ease, plenty of energy, and without stopping.

When you get up out of a chair and start somewhere, even to the mailbox or bathroom, begin breathing as you walk. Deep breathing not only helps your circulation, it feeds oxygen to every cell through the bloodstream, combats poisons in the body, and increases mental alertness. So make a daily habit of breathing deeply. If you don't have time or inclination to count, merely breathe deeply and often throughout the day.

My own favorite breathing method for situations like these is to breathe in deeply, then exhale through the mouth like a soundless whistle.

The book mentioned in the previous chapter, *Yoga for People Over 50,* by Suza Norton, gives some exciting results of Yoga breathing as well as easy-to-follow directions on how to do it. Here are some of the impressive things this excellent and helpful book says about breathing:

"Most people, young and old, use only one-third of their breathing capacity. . . . This continuous inadequate supply of oxygen to the body accelerates the aging process, gradually impairing the functioning of vital organs."

"Through the years slouching in chairs, overeating, work, and other tensions prohibit the complete and efficient use of the lungs."

"Slow, even, complete breathing is more conducive to a feeling of vitality than almost any other single factor."

"When you learn to slow down your breathing consciously, there is less wear and tear on the entire body—less work for the heart, lower blood pressure, and a general soothing of body tensions."

"Breathing habits are really easier to change than eating habits, but just as important to your health."

You really owe it to yourself to read and apply the information in this book to help you breathe properly, which is a giant step toward rejuvenation.

### A New "Find"

One of the world's greatest fears is aging. People will succumb to any advertising, any gadget, any product, even surgery, if it will promise them protection from aging. Actually, there is no single panacea for aging (with the possible exception of one approach I will describe in the last chapter). So do not allow yourself to be gullible about it.

There are, however, various honest methods that may help. I have included them in this book. I refuse to discuss or even mention anything that might conceivably be a hoax, or a con game, and thus another disappointment to a person who tries something with great hope, only to find it is a dud or a "rip-off."

I have recently found something new, which I have spent much time in researching and which I feel has promise. In fact I am using it myself. Laboratory tests show that it can help people at any age, particularly those in later life. This "find" is a machine known as a "negative ionizer."

In certain parts of the world at various times certain types of winds blow that cause all manner of discomfort—mentally, emotionally, and physically. People may become irritable, even violent or suicidal, under the influence of these winds. There is the *Foehn* in Germany and Switzerland; the *Mistral* in southern France; the *Hamsin* in the Middle East; the *Chinook* in the Pacific Northwest of the United States; and the *Santa Ana* in southern California.

The effects of these winds on people can be so disastrous that some doctors refuse to operate just before or during the time they are blowing, and judges are more lenient toward crimes and the increase of traffic accidents occurring at such times.

Years of study finally revealed that these winds produce electrical charges known as positive ions, which seem to be responsible for the disturbances felt by people. When the winds cease and the atmosphere is tranquil again, negative ions take over and calm is restored.

As a result of this scientific research, negative ionizing machines, after having been banned over twenty years ago because of claims benefiting a long list of physical and emotional disorders, are again becoming available. You cannot keep a good thing down forever, however, and the negative ionizers are back on the market, but with the warning to manufacturers that they must be called air cleansers, about which no medical claims are allowed.

Before I tell you the list of disorders negative ions are reported to helped, you may have experienced them yourself in nature. There are high concentrations of negative ions on mountaintops, as well as close to the beach where the waves crash. A waterfall or running, splashing shower can produce negative ions. It is interesting that some of the longest-lived, healthiest centenarians live in mountain villages. The best most of us can do is to vacation in the high mountains or relax on the beach near the waves during an annual vacation. A negative ionizer changes all this. You can have the ions in your own home at the twist of a dial.

What do the ionizers accomplish? I will list below the benefits reported, with their sources. This is strictly *reporting* and in no way intended to make medical claims.

Negative ions have been helpful for:
—tranquilizing and insomnia
—hay fever, bronchitis, sinus, asthma, and emphysema
—depression, tension, even suicidal tendencies
—use in hospitals for speeding healing of postoperative conditions as well as burns
—aching joints
—fatigue

—delivery of more oxygen to various tissues of the body (so necessary to the aging), with improved mental efficiency and many other benefits.

No danger or side effects from natural or machine-made negative ions have ever been found.

You may contend that you do not live in an area where winds producing high positive ions blow. Perhaps not. But positive ions can be generated by other causes in our environment than these disturbing winds. Air conditioning and machinery, such as cars and planes, can generate positive ions leading to positive ion poisoning. So can synthetic fabrics in clothes, carpets, and furnishings, as well as cigarette smoke.

I turn my ionizer on in my bedroom and sleep with it running (it is quiet) *every* night, *all* night. A friend of mine who suffers from emphysema wrote me recently that he detected no improvement in his chest condition after using the ionizer. "But," he added, "I do not remember to turn it on except occasionally." No wonder! Until symptoms are under control, the effect of an ionizer is noticeable only after continuous use, not a now-and-then use. As an extra bonus, my ionizer completely cleans the air in my room three times every hour and does away with household or cooking odors in a very short time. I am now planning to buy a portable ionizer to carry with me in my car or in transit when I travel by other means.

WHERE TO OBTAIN NEGATIVE IONIZERS (OR AIR CLEANSERS)

Amron, Ltd., Industrial Zone, Herzlya "B," P.O. Box 336, Israel (These are imported into the U.S. at present. One

Israel-made ionizer, known as Modulion, is available from San Rafael Health Foods, 1132 Fourth Avenue, San Rafael, California 94901.)
Dev Industries, Inc., 5721 Arapahoe, Boulder, Colorado 80302
Medion, Ltd., Box 1, Oxted, Surrey, England
Multorgan, S.A., CH 6893, Magliaso, Lugano, Switzerland
Santek, Inc., P.O. Box 6036, Hollywood, Florida 33021
*Please write to the distributors (not to me) for information and prices.*

### SOURCES OF INFORMATION ABOUT NEGATIVE IONIZERS

1. Hal Aigner, "Positive Effects from Negative Ions," *Pacific Sun*, November 11–17, 1977
2. Albert Paul Krueger, M.D., Professor Emeritus of Biometeorology, University of California, Berkeley, and Eddie James Reed, "Biological Impact of Small Air Ions," *Science*, September 2, 1976, Vol. 193, pp. 1209–13
3. Robert O'Brien, "Ions Can Do Strange Things to You," *The Reader's Digest*, October, 1960
4. Fred Soyka, with Alan Edmonds, *The Ion Effect.* New York: E.P. Dutton & Co., 1977 (a fascinating, informative, and readable book)

# 15

## Changing Your Life
## Through Thought

FEELING LEFT OUT, or on your own, or ignored by others is sometimes a Senior's own fault. It is always easier to blame others for your misfortune than to face up to your own weaknesses. But at this time of life it is crucial to set up your new way of life in such a way that you attract others instead of repelling them.

Because many aging people may be depressed at the death of a mate, or loss of a job or status of some kind—or because they may have let their health slip and do not feel well—they become cranky, crotchety, rigid, complaining, faultfinding, instead of flexible. Obviously this is not the route to popularity. Such negative attitudes scare away everybody except those who are forced to stand by to care for the aging person, whereas they would rather flee or hide.

But there are also parents who act like martyrs, believing that since they gave their all to their children, their children should give their all to them. Worse yet is the parent left behind by the death of a mate, who transfers dependence from a departed husband or wife and clings to or commandeers their children, preventing them from making a life of their own. If these juniors try to achieve independence, the parent, perhaps unconsciously, stages a rage, pours out tears of recrimination, or manages a heart attack or some other psychosomatic ailment to obtain the abject submission of a son or daughter or a whole family of children.

I know an attractive, highly successful professio. woman who lost her husband by death. She has substituted her son in many ways for the departed husband. The son is required to wait on her hand and foot, give up his own friends and interests in order to serve his mother's demands according to her constantly changing whims.

Another overlooked fault in many Seniors is not having anything to look forward to. All too often they live in the past, monopolizing the conversation with accounts of past deeds and successes, even old jokes, repeating them again and again to the intense boredom of any captive audience. This, of course, is due to lack of attention or a feeling of insecurity on the part of the Senior, who is trying to shore up his or her own ego or status that has slipped. Obviously, this habit can alienate everyone within earshot.

Fortunately, not all Seniors are so thoughtless or selfish. Nor do they need to be. Better to be cheerful, develop a pleasant sense of humor, be a good listener, and show genuine interest in the problems of others. As a result, friends and relatives can be attracted to them as bees to honey, even though these same Seniors may be suffering emotionally. Wisely, they have decided that there is nothing to be gained by unloading their sorrows on others or wallowing in self-pity. So they have deliberately substituted a cheerful façade to present to the public. Even people who are pain-ridden or blind have proved to be highly popular, full of infectious good spirits, so that they cheer up those who need it. The secret here is that these individuals are full of love for others instead of self-love, are never critical or complaining. They thereby acquire charm and are beloved by others. Just remember that there is always some good in everyone if you look for it. Do not let anyone leave your presence without saying something good about whoever it may be. As has been said: "Give him roses before he dies; don't wait until afterward; then it is too late."

And do you know what? Persons who started out as disagreeable and deliberately acted agreeable have eventually *become* agreeable! This is because they have programmed their computer, which is giving out what they put into it.

Scientists have recently discovered a breakthrough in the control of the mind over the body. It is so rewarding that it can become the most fascinating game you ever played. You can get anything you want if you just learn the rules of how to program your computer correctly. You can be well instead of sick, happy instead of sad, vital and energetic instead of weak, and wealthy instead of poor. There is practically no limit except for possibly not being able to grow a new limb. But you can program your life so that it is better than ever before.

I could write a book full of other examples of people who have done it, but I'll give you one quick example before telling you how you can do it too.

One woman I am proud to call a friend is in her late

seventies. She has been widowed, endured much suffering, including several near-fatal ailments. Yet she
devotes her life to helping others, is now happily mar-
ried to her second husband, is surrounded by countless admirers, who are so attracted to her that they follow her wherever she goes, basking in her radiance
and love, which she bestows on all alike. She is truly
beautiful inside and out. This adulation is deserved,
because she has earned it through her own efforts to
forget herself and help others unselfishly with their
problems.

In order to change your life for the better through
thought control the secret is that our subconscious
mind soaks up, without logic or reasoning, whatever
we think and feel, right or wrong. It acts exactly as a
computer, putting out what is put into it. If you think
sickness, sooner or later your subconscious will attract it! If you think poverty, the same thing happens.
But if you think health or happiness *consistently,* that
is what will become manifest, sooner or later. You can
depend upon it.

You may say, "Oh, I've tried that. It doesn't work
for me." The reason may be that you decided to be
cheerful for one day and let sadness take over the
next. Your computer (the subconscious) first gets the
message "cheer," then, just as it is getting to work to
follow instructions, you give it a countermessage of
"sadness," which cancels out the first message. This
jams the works, and nothing at all happens! In other
words, *you are what you think.* But there is a little trick
here: You can add feeling to speed the action of the
subconscious, as well as supply a visualization blueprint picturing whatever you wish (which shouldn't be

changed every ten minutes or every day). You may have to fake the feeling you desire at first and try to feel healthy or cheerful even if you aren't. Pretty soon the idea will be picked up by your subconscious slave, and it will do your bidding.

Here is an example of another friend.

She too is radiant, joyful, happy, and loving, and attracts unlimited friends and followers. But I was surprised when she told me she was not always that way. She has had one of the most tragic lives I ever heard of, but she suddenly realized that the negative conditions in her life were not improving, but worsening. So one day she made a firm decision: From that day forward she would not think a negative thought or speak a negative word, no matter how strong the temptation.

It was not an easy changeover. The subconscious does not like change and becomes grumpy, trying to pull you back into your old ways, because it is an easier, lazier way. But my friend, who is in her late sixties, was determined. Soon the fight was over, and she had won. Through constructive thinking she made herself *feel* cheerful and happy, though just the opposite was true at first. What could the subconscious computer do, other than balk, but obey? Sometimes you have to get pretty stern with your subconscious and talk to it in no uncertain terms. Many people give their subconscious a name, like Charles or Vivian. You may have to say firmly, "Now listen, George, stop this nonsense. I want action NOW! I want you to . . . ," giving the command you expect to have followed. You may have to do it at least three times at one sitting to make sure the message gets through; and if you are not wishy-washy, but firm, it *will* get through.

At any rate, the affairs of my friend began to turn in the right direction. After being tragically widowed twice, she now attracted an adoring mate, and in many other ways she is truly happy, one of the best examples of computing I know.

In addition to consistent input of ideas, firmness, and feeling the way you want to feel (even though the desired condition hasn't yet manifested), the subconscious also likes pictures. It helps get the idea across faster. I have tried this myself many times with surprising results.

For example, I may have a desk piled high with unanswered letters I dread doing, so I use the visualization method. I form a picture of the desk clean as a whistle, seeing myself feeling happy that I have finished the job. Then I put it out of my mind and forget it. (A watched pot never boils.) Some time later, when I least expect it, I suddenly feel just like doing the job, and turn to it with eagerness. In no time, it seems, it has gone speedily without any hang-ups, and the job is done. My desk is as clear as I envisioned it, and I feel as happy as I had wished.

This can be done with health too. You can visualize yourself looking and feeling well until you *do* feel well. Don't dwell on it or how it will come about in the meantime; this only delays it. Let the subconscious know what is needed and ask it to bring it to you. I never cease to marvel at what can happen. Sometimes I find that I may need a certain food or vitamin or something else to help my progress. It often takes time for the subconscious to discover this and bring it to you. But keep at it and the necessary help will come.

Warning: If you are not sure that something is right

for you—let's say a certain job, or a mate, or a house—you had better qualify your demand with the statement, "according to the will of God," or you might get something you later wished you hadn't.

One of the most helpful booklets I have ever read on this subject of computing is called *Key to Yourself*, by the late Dr. Venice Bloodworth, a trained counselor in helping others, who testified that her "computing" method changed their lives. I am going to share some of the helpful statements in this book, which has already sold fifteen printings to delighted readers. Dr. Bloodworth wrote:

"Like attracts like. Whatever you hold in mind any length of time MUST come into expression for you."

"Some people reap what they sow: failure— because they do not stick to their goal. Decide what you want and stick to it."

"To have health, you must concentrate on health; to be loved, you must first love others; to have abundance, you must think abundance. Ignore the present conditions and hold fast to your new mental picture."

She urges you to concentrate on what you want, *not on what you don't want*. Thoughts of discord, worry, envy, fear will be set in motion, sooner or later, bringing on those exact conditions. You cannot afford to harbor them for a minute! Don't forget, too, to avoid fear of *anything*. Since this is a magnetic *feeling*, as the Bible says, "What you fear will come upon you." But so will any other strong positive feeling bring *good* results. As Dr. Bloodworth concludes: "The magic secret of attainment is intense desire. Fix one goal at a time and concentrate on it exclusively."

You can use little helps to keep up your courage

while the changes you have computed are going through the incubation stage, before they appear. No doubt you remember that old motto of Coué: "Every day in every way I am getting better and better." It has worked for thousands who have used it consistently.

You can amend this to suit your needs, and chant it to yourself as you walk: "Every day in every way I am getting healthier and healthier," or "I am becoming healthy, youthful, and loving," or whatever you wish. Just press the right word button with force and repetition, and you can reshape your life as you want it to be.

# 16

## Helps for Special Senior Problems

### *Your Feet*

SINCE zones on the bottoms of your feet reflect areas throughout the entire body, it is not surprising that when your feet ache, you may ache all over. There are books on reflexology[1, 2] to help you learn what is wrong with your feet as well as your body. Not only can you locate clues on the bottoms of your feet, but even though you do not have a book or foot chart, here is what you can do to obtain relief:

Explore, with your fingers, every inch of the bottoms of both feet, even under and around your toes, pressing firmly as you go. When you locate a sore spot, this is a sign of foot congestion, also linked to some congested area in the body. For example, your liver, or kidney, and other organs and glands are represented in some spot (or nerve ending) on your feet.

To correct, for a few seconds every day gently massage the sore spots with your fingertips to help break up the congestion until the soreness disappears. You may be surprised at the results, though they are not necessarily instantaneous. You will see by case histories in some of the books on the subject that many people have experienced near-miracles through reflexology.

How many women, after a shopping tour, can hardly wait to get home to kick off their shoes? That is probably because they are wearing the wrong type of shoes. We shudder at the Orientals who formerly bound the feet of their women to keep them small and dainty. But we think nothing of trying to squeeze our own feet into shoes manufactured for the "average" person.

I recently read of a young man with one foot size 10 and the other foot size 8 1/2 who could not get one pair of shoes to fit both feet, so he took to making his own shoes for comfort. Nearly all of us have one foot larger, yet the smaller foot slides around in the size chosen to fit the larger foot, or the larger foot is constricted by the smaller size for vanity's sake. As for platform soles and heels, or stiletto heels, they can be forms of torture. The spine and posture are tipped out of alignment, and the whole body, as well as the feet, suffers. What area reflects this suffering first? Your face! No wonder our young people are rebelling and reverting to bare feet or sandals.

Fortunately, there are a few ready-made "natural shoes" available today. Some people prefer one type; others like another. My favorite, and apparently many Californians agree with me, is called the *Birkenstock* footprint sandal, which feels as if you are making your own footprints in wet sand. The blessed relief that comes from wearing these sandals is almost incredible. Leg aches, backaches, foot aches have disappeared in men and women, and a feeling of buoyancy results.

The footprint sandal is not pretty, but it is beginning to be considered "smart." You can wear it for walking, working, gardening, shopping, and casual wear, and reserve your dress shoes for special occasions only. I could not manage without mine. *Birkenstocks* are made in Germany, but available in the U.S. (see Product List for source), and no more expensive than ordinary dress shoes. And oh, what comfort! One pair outlasts several pairs of cheaper, shoddier sandals.

## *Leg and Other Cramps*

People of all ages often become frightened when they suffer from leg cramps. Except for swimming cramps, a cramp is usually nothing more serious than a mild deficiency of certain nutrients and can soon be corrected permanently, perhaps in several days, so that it will not return.

The most common cause of leg or other cramps in the extremities is a shortage of calcium. These cramps may occur in the legs at night, and in the hands, fingers, or even in the upper ribs (where they may be mistaken for a heart attack) during the day.

Taking sufficient calcium may still not rid you of the cramps if it is not assimilated. Vitamin D (400 units a day in tablet form) is needed for calcium assimilation. Or a lack of acid in the system can also cause cramps. Calcium needs acid to dissolve it in the bloodstream so that it can be properly assimilated instead of piling up in the joints, where it is not wanted. Those who drink quantities of milk for calcium may still be deficient, since milk calcium may not be properly assimilated as one grows older. A surer way is to take calcium lactate or calcium gluconate tablets (available at drug and health stores). These forms of calcium are among the easiest to assimilate. But check your acid intake too. If necessary, add HCL to your diet, or sip apple cider vinegar in water to taste with your meals. Too much lecithin, taken over a prolonged period, can also produce a calcium deficiency and result in cramps. This is because lecithin is rich in phosphorus, which has a close affinity for calcium and is excreted with it from the body. The solution is not to avoid lecithin, a superior product, but to increase the calcium intake to make up for the deficit if you find you are having leg or other cramps.

A deficiency of B$_6$ has also been known to cause the Charley-horse type of cramps in the calves of the legs.

If a cramp attacks while you are in bed, lie on your back and point your toes toward the ceiling until the cramp passes. If this fails, stand or walk on your feet, or get into a tub of warm water. Meanwhile, start correcting your dietary deficiency—the amount of calcium you need to take depends on individual results—and you will soon be delivered of the cramps.

### Smoking

As you know, smoking has been found medically to be a definite cause of lung cancer. But there are other hazards you may not know of. Smoking can also lead to faster aging. Smoking has even led to heart attacks, not only in smokers themselves, but in those toward whom smokers blow their smoke! Researchers have found also that smoking definitely causes facial wrinkles. It may be a matter of time, but if you continue smoking, those wrinkles will come.

Some people smoke because they are shy, nervous, insecure, or under stress. They may also be victims of hypoglycemia, due to dietary lack of protein and B vitamins, as well as too many sweets.

I will share with you a method Captain William P. Knowles (mentioned in the chapter on breathing) has developed. He says that of his students, from a hundred countries, eight out of ten have stopped smoking entirely or greatly reduced their intake by this method. One secretary, who smoked twenty-five cigarettes daily and had suffered from bronchitis and a cough, stopped smoking in two months. Later she tried a cigarette to test herself. She said the taste was awful. Her desire to smoke had disappeared, together with the bronchitis and the cough.

Here is Captain Knowles's method for stopping the smoking habit. It is done three times daily for three minutes each time.

1. Sit upright in a chair. Don't touch the back of the chair with your spine.

2. Stretch your arms forward, then draw them back slowly; let your elbows rest against the sides of your body; put hands, palms down, on your thighs.

3. Breathe in and out quickly through your nose about a dozen times. A smoker may cough and sputter, but this is good for expelling phlegm and stale air.

4. Once the lungs are cleansed, exhale slowly and completely until there is no air left in your lungs. Then inhale to the count of seven. Pause for one second,

then exhale. Do this breathing fourteen times, seven in and seven out. Keep your chest out and shoulders back to allow freedom for breathing. That's it!

An excellent book showing the social-physical hazards of smoking is Don C. Matchan's paperback, *We Mind If You Smoke.*

## Constipation

People spend more time worrying about constipation than necessary. It is easily conquered once you learn how. Laxatives are not the answer for two reasons: They flush out of the body your water soluble vitamin/mineral intake by drawing on the body fluids to produce an evacuation. They are also habit forming, so that you become dependent on them.

If you have an emergency, herbal laxatives from health stores are safer than commercial products or taking *any* laxative daily. A cup of yogurt, or a teaspoon of whole flaxseed or powdered psyllium seed swallowed quickly with water (the seeds become gelatinous once swallowed) will usually tide you over your immediate difficulty.

My favorite is clay. If you have not read that wonderful book, *Our Earth, Our Cure,* by Raymond Dextreit, explaining what certain clays can do for you, you have missed something. I have never known anyone who read this book who didn't rave about it.

There are various clays, and some are better for different purposes, some for external, others for internal use. The one I use is imported from France, green clay, loaded with minerals, and a surefire, natural, easy remedy for constipation. You stir up one teaspoonful of it in a half-glass of water and let it sit all day or all night. (Do *not* leave the metal spoon in the glass.) In the morning, or at night, drink the water that remains at the top after the clay has settled. Depending upon your needs, take it either before breakfast or before bedtime (it works about eight hours later), or, as many people do, take it both times. It also acts as a detoxifier and gives you many added benefits. (See Product List for the source.)

The most popular constipation remedy at the present time is a high-fiber diet. This means plenty of fresh raw fruits and vegetables. Or, if it agrees with you, you can take bran. The bran should not be rough and scratchy, but in softer flake form. Taken together with plenty of water, bran swells to provide bulk, and doctors and laymen are happy with the results. You can take a teaspoon as a starter for a few days and then increase as necessary. It can also be sprinkled over cereals, raw or or cooked. At my house I make my own bran muffins. Here is the recipe. They are excellent for breakfast. Everybody likes them.

## BRAN MUFFINS

*Mixture One*

In a bowl combine:
1 cup unbleached flour
1 cup bran flakes (from health store)
3 teaspoons baking powder
1 cup blueberries, fresh or frozen, or other fruit of your choice. Or you may use raisins or chopped dates, plus spices. Experiment with variations. (Choose any amount you wish.)

*Mixture Two*

In a blender, or other container, combine:
1 cup milk
Honey to taste (I use approximately 1/4 cup)
1 egg
3 tablespoons oil

Stir each mixture well and separately, then combine the two. Stir, do not beat, until the batter is well blended. It should be stiff. If not, add more bran, or flour, or both. Drop by spoonfuls into a greased muffin pan, or crinkled paper cups inserted into pan (to avoid scrubbing the pan afterward). Bake at 400° until lightly brown (about thirty minutes). Makes a dozen muffins.

Eat one or two daily, according to your needs. Leftovers can be moistened and reheated in a slightly warm oven. Or they can be split and toasted.

## *Insomnia*

There is nothing more aggravating than not being able to sleep. But sleeping pills are NOT the answer. They can become habit forming and are also potentially dangerous. Combined with alcohol they can be as fatal as if you gulped down too many. Why take a chance when there are easier, safer methods?

Adelle Davis recommended keeping calcium (lactate) tablets on your bedside table. She called them lullaby pills. She said if you need more during the night, take them. They are harmless.

Personally, I keep on my bedside table something I like better: the small homeopathic specific cell salt tablets for such problems. You dissolve them dry on the

tongue. If you cannot sleep, take approximately a teaspoon of these tiny tablets, and they will soon send
you to dreamland. They are called *Nerve Tonic Tablets*, are available at health stores, and absolutely safe
and nonhabit forming. Others prefer a combination of
these same "cell salts," plus herbs, called *Calms
Forté*. Health stores say they cannot keep this popular
remedy in stock. These two latter products can also be
useful for stressful situations.

Getting more exercise daily may help you sleep better at night. Outdoor workers rarely suffer from insomnia.

What you eat before you go to bed influences your
sleeping too. Often the later you eat before bedtime,
the harder you will find it to sleep restfully, without
tossing, turning, and bad dreams. Adelle Davis always
recommended a large breakfast, a medium lunch, and
a light "supper." This was found to promote better
sleeping, as proved by a study done in a California
prison back in the 1930's. This study found that the
more protein taken just before bedtime, the greater the
sleep disturbance. Fats or carbohydrates seemed preferable, and eating less or nothing at all near bedtime
produced the least restlessness of all. However, some
people who eat lightly or not at all in the evening may
wake up hungry in the middle of the night, so use your
own judgment.

Certain types of mild exercise taken just before bedtime can help overcome insomnia. One doctor, Ed-
mund Jacobsen, M.D., a relaxation specialist, suggests relaxing your eye and throat muscles as you go to
sleep. He has found that this hastens sleep more
quickly than relaxing any other part of your body.

Another doctor, M. N. Pai, recommends our Muscle Massage technique, described in Chapter 13, to induce all-over body relaxation.

Try counting your blessings instead of sheep, and if you simply cannot sleep, don't lie there; get up and do a boring chore until you do feel sleepy.

Although eight hours of sleep have been recommended for the average person, this may or may not apply to everybody. There has been some speculation that the older a person becomes, the less sleep is needed. The Russians, supported by their scientific research in this area, refute this, believing that one hour of sleep for every three of the twenty-four-hour day— or eight hours—can regenerate cells and metabolism, particularly of the aging individual. Without this amount of sleep they believe that normal, daily activity can destroy the cells and metabolism faster than they can be rebuilt.

As proof they cite the well-documented dog study. An old dog had lost all of his teeth, and his coat sadly lacked the luster of youth. He was checked continuously during a three-months' experiment in rejuvenation by a staff of doctors and technicians in the laboratory. During this time the dog was kept asleep, by means of a harmless drug, twenty-three out of twenty-four hours daily and was given vitamins, minerals, proteins, and other food supplements in concentrated form by intravenous injections. After the sixth week a change took place in the dog. His coat became soft and glossy, and he appeared younger. At the end of twelve weeks (the end of the experiment) he was playing like a puppy and looking and acting young.

Even though man's life span is six times longer than

a dog's, and it might take man six times longer for similar rejuvenation, the experimenters believe that through extra sleep, as well as extra nutrients, cells are rebuilt and metabolism is restimulated faster than activity could destroy them. (This study was conducted by Dr. Baines at the Davidovsky Laboratory, U.S.S.R. Psychiatry Institute, in 1957.)

### Overweight and Fasting

I have written a small book on this problem. It is called *Be Slim* and *Healthy*, and it has all of the safe answers for reducing. A recent tip: When you discover that most carbohydrates are the weight-makers, do NOT avoid fresh fruits. They are high in carbohydrates, but you can lose weight on them because they contain enzymes. (This information arrived after I had finished the book.) Otherwise, everything you want to know about losing weight safely, without hunger and without fasting (which I disapprove of), is included in the book just mentioned. It is in paperback at health stores.

### Acid-Alkaline Balance

This subject is so greatly misunderstood that I have refused to tackle it before. Some foods, which seem to be acid, produce in your body an alkaline reaction, and some foods and vegetables, which seem to be nonacid, produce acid. It is very confusing. Let's simplify it once and for all. Citrus fruits, which taste like acid, actually can produce alkalinity. Lemon juice is less of a problem. Since it is so sour, most people do not take too much of it. But people who guzzle orange or grapefruit juice think they are doing themselves a favor, partly because they are told these juices contain vitamin C. You have to drink a lot of these juices to get the amount of vitamin C in one 250 or 500 mg. tablet. Vitamin C or apple cider vinegar can provide acid in a helpful form. Judge Tom R. Blaine, in his book *Goodbye Allergies* (a Nutri-book in paperback published by the Kensington Publishing Corporation, 521 Fifth Avenue, New York, N.Y. 10017), says: "Taking excessive amounts of citrus and other juices over a long period of time may produce an alkalyzed system, indicated by nasal [and anal] itching, as well as headaches, restlessness, and inability to sleep."

Most people need more acid-promoting foods than alkaline foods. Just remember this: *A germ cannot live in an acid medium.* In the laboratory germs are grown in an alkaline medium, which may be sugars or other forms of alkalinity. But they are killed by acid.

Sometimes, if you find yourself feeling very weary or prone to any germ that comes along, try some apple cider vinegar in water and sip it with your meals (or between meals) like wine. You will feel a pickup in minutes. It is similar to turning on the electricity that lights up the room. Acid apparently generates body electricity. Make your own apple cider vinegar mixture to taste pleasant, and see for yourself. It mixes well with honey.

### Alcohol

Avoid hard liquors. I have covered this subject thoroughly in my *Handbook of Natural Remedies for Common Ailments*, so I will not repeat it here. Suffice to say that Seniors who do not have anything pleasant to look forward to may often enjoy a 3-ounce glass of dry wine (preferably red) just prior to, or with, the evening meal. No more! You can become a "wino" as easily as a hard-drinking alcoholic, so use this treat according to the rules instead of abusing it.

## *Teeth and Gums*

One problem that plagues Seniors is diminishing or weakening teeth, as well as gum afflictions. There is a nutritional remedy for these problems, and the sooner you begin, the quicker the results. The remedies are nutritional, and need time to be built into your body. They work well, but are not instantaneous.

Calcium is an integral part of our bones and teeth. If we do not get enough calcium, then one part of the body borrows it from another part, often from the teeth, causing cavities. Also, as we have said before, there may be a sufficient calcium intake, but if there is insufficient acid to digest it, the calcium merely piles up in unwanted places without doing the job it is supposed to do.

Seniors who develop loose teeth will be cheered by a study conducted by two Cornell University researchers. When 1,000 mgs. of calcium gluconate or calcium carbonate were given patients *on a daily basis for six months*, X-rays showed that fresh bone had appeared in the jaw bones (which hold teeth firm).[3]

Bone meal, especially raw bone meal, is particularly helpful in rebuilding bones, preventing or speeding the healing of fractures, sometimes arresting cavities, even repairing them in some cases and *preventing frac-*

*tures.* (Seniors are prone to fractures.) I fed my mother bone meal every day of her life from age sixty on until she died at eighty-seven. She did not suffer a single fracture, although many of her contemporaries did. (Bone meal is available at health stores in tablet or powdered form.)

As for gum disturbances, vitamin C, as well as Bioflavonoids (the entire C complex or family), firms up gums and prevents or heals weak and bleeding gums. But there is a substance, advocated in the Edgar Cayce readings, called *Ipsab* that stops bleeding and heals gums almost overnight (see Product List).

### Appearance

There is no reason for Seniors to look unattractive. You can be attractive at any age, and you should be, to give others as well as yourself pleasure. No one likes to see a droopy, unpleasant-looking person.

As an example, a true story recently appeared in a newspaper of a woman who decided to test this idea. She wore her worst-looking jeans, left off her makeup, and let her hair become tousled and uncombed. Attired in the most unattractive way possible, she entered a bank and asked to cash a fifty-dollar check. The bank refused, saying she did not have an account there. She was treated coolly and without respect.

Next she went to a good restaurant and asked for a table. She was hastily hidden behind a large plant, where she waited while forty other customers, though they came in later than she, were seated ahead of her.

Next she went to an expensive dress shop and was told she could not try on dresses unless she was clean.

Two days later the same woman, her hair well groomed, her makeup artfully applied, and her clothes neat and attractive, went into the same bank, asked to cash another fifty-dollar check, and got the cash immediately.

In the same restaurant as before she was promptly given an excellent table. And at the same dress shop as before she was encouraged to try on thousand-dollar dresses (actually she had only thirty dollars in her wallet).

So looks do count!

### *And a Note of Advice to Grown Children and Well-meaning Friends*

Today it is rare to find a younger person, particularly in the early and later teen-age group, who wouldn't rather be caught dead than even be seen conversing with an older adult. Listen to the elders. Let them talk, at least *try* to be interested in their problems and interests. And don't be condescending. Treat them normally, not like children.

And for those grown children who have elderly friends or parents, do not drop in on them without warning. No one in the older age group wants to be embarrassed by being caught without such props as contact lenses (they may not be able to see you well), or a hearing aid (they may not hear what you are saying), or their false teeth (without which they may appear frightening). You may say, "How silly, why let a little thing like that upset you?" Don't judge prematurely. Most of us want to put our best face forward. Wait until you are your parents' age. Don't judge glibly or thoughtlessly. Most people are very sensitive about not appearing "normal."

One friend's husband had had his leg amputated below the knee. He has an artificial leg, but like other artificial spare parts, even false teeth, it is often very uncomfortable to wear these substitutes hour in, hour out. This man, when he had donned his new leg and put on his trousers, after long, hard, painful hours of adjusting to it, had learned to walk so well that few people knew of his handicap. Yet at home, when only his wife is present, due to discomfort, he does not put on the device until necessary. He lives in dread of someone dropping in unannounced and catching him without his substitute leg. I unthinkingly dropped in one day without previous announcement. I heard scurrying noises behind the door after I rang the bell, then his wife answered the door looking a bit flurried. I immediately asked for her husband, and she explained with embarrassment that he was in the other room hastily putting on his artificial leg.

With older people in particular thoughtfulness goes a long way in helping them see—and thus feel—themselves in the best light.

For guidance in improving your appearance, read the next chapter carefully.

### REFERENCES
(See *Bibliography* for fuller details.)

1. Mildred Carter, *Helping Yourself to Foot Reflexology.*
2. Anna Kaye, with Don C. Matcham, *Mirror of the Body.*
3. Linda Clark, *Know Your Nutrition.*

# 17

## How to Improve Your
## Appearance at Any Age

THERE IS NO excuse these days to accept defeat about your appearance. You can always improve it, no matter what your age or sex. Although much of the information I am about to share with you is intended for women, there are helpful hints here men too can use. Since it has long been no secret that husbands dip into their wives' cosmetics on occasion, now cosmetics are being made for men too.

There are many beauty publications available that will help you enhance your appearance in your mature years to its fullest, loveliest, or handsomest. For instance, the little paperback, *Beauty Questions and Answers*, by Linda Clark and her daughter Karen Kelly, a beauty columnist, is packed with tips about how to do it on your own. Another source book is Linda Clark's earlier classic, *Secrets of Health and Beauty*, now an international winner. Another approach to self-

*This chapter was contributed by Betty Franklin, consultant for Beauty Naturally, Inc.*

rejuvenation techniques is provided in the book, *Health, Youth and Beauty through Color Breathing,* by Linda Clark and Yvonne Martine. In this book is the exciting story of a woman who actually turned back the clock for herself and others by a unique method.

Now for some specific means to enhance your appearance.

One unfailing help is using a slant board a few minutes each day, with head lower than feet to encourage fresh circulation to face, scalp, and neck. As blood flow is stimulated, so is oxygenation, needed to remove waste products from our bodies and produce sparkle in eyes, face, and brain.

The slant board reverses the downward pull of gravity and so helps to diminish wrinkles and droopy muscles in face and neck. It is also restful and refreshing. Just a few minutes on the slant board helps you to look more relaxed and rested, and because your facial muscles have been pulled *up* instead of down, you will look younger. Serenity is a great beautifier too, and the slant board encourages it. Try lying on it while listening to restful music.

If you do not have a slant board, you can easily make one. Get a wide board from the lumber yard, or even use your own ironing board, raising the foot-end fifteen inches on bricks, or you can simply lie comfortably on your back on your bed, with pillows under your hips and your feet elevated on books or pillows.

One note of caution, however: If you have circulatory problems, at first lie on the board only a few minutes and get up very slowly. As you get used to this upended position, you can remain on the board longer and eventually get up more easily. You will soon adjust to the sudden increase of circulation to your head, and lose the "swimmy-headed" feeling on arising. Meanwhile, the rewards of lying on a slant board are great. Early psychological tests made with students at Colgate University showed that the brain was more active and alert after a siesta on the slant board. So men as well as women can benefit.

Appearance can be improved for both men and women by doing face exercises. The principle here is that the face, as well as the body, needs exercise to tone up muscles. Also, a shortened muscle does not droop, and exercises do shorten as well as strengthen muscles. There are several books on face exercises available: an inexpensive one by Linda Clark[1] and an excellent and slightly more expensive one by Senta Maria Rungé.[2] My own favorite is one written by Dr. Robert Alan Franklyn called *Shiatsu—60 Minutes to Facial Beauty* (published by Doctor Beauty, Inc., Publications, 8760 Sunset Blvd., Los Angeles, California 90067). Dr. Franklyn is an internationally known cosmetic surgeon, and his system of face exercises employs the technique of Japanese finger pressure on certain facial points similar to acupressure points. This, in turn, he finds, stimulates circulation and revitalizes tissues. These exercises are quick and easy to do. I use them to "wake up" my own face every morning.

## Should You Have a Face-Lift?

Perhaps you've been thinking that cosmetic surgery would be the next best thing to finding the fountain of youth, at least temporarily. Certainly, despite the enormous cost involved, this approach to rejuvenation is a way of life nowadays. In fact, even young persons begin having tucks and lifts at the first sign of a wrinkle, bag, or sag. But as the old saying goes, "All that glitters is not gold." There are serious considerations involved.

I have repeatedly heard reputable surgeons advise people to keep the following aspects in mind before deciding on cosmetic repair: (1) Make certain you select a fully qualified specialist. Evidently there are charlatans in the business, who butcher rather than enhance. (2) Surgery always involves possible risks, regardless of the surgeon's skill. (3) Healing can be very slow in some cases, particularly if a person is not in top condition. (4) A face-lift can't be expected to bring about miraculous changes in lifestyle and attitudes, yours or those of others toward you. (5) Actually, if your looks are altered too drastically, there can be problems and disappointment.

I know both men and women who were convinced their appearance was causing all their troubles and finally resorted to cosmetic surgery, only to discover that the change didn't make any difference at all. In fact, sometimes changed features have caused frustration and confusion. People have told me they "just didn't feel like themselves" anymore. In other instances, however, some changes have been remarkably successful. So it's important to weigh all pros and cons before deciding to invest in such a luxury, which is, at best, temporary. If you're convinced it would make you happy, even for a few years, good luck!

However, I hope you'll consider the alternatives discussed in this chapter. Remember, first of all, that correct nutrition, if consistent, can improve skin and muscle tone to a remarkable degree. So can specific exercises, which some plastic surgeons advocate both to prevent the need for face-lifts and to help maintain muscle integrity after surgery.

Recently, a makeup expert from one of the largest cosmetic houses in the world reported that photographs taken of women who had had cosmetic surgery were no better than those of women who had learned corrective makeup for their individual problems from an expert cosmetician. In other words, there *appeared* to be no visible difference between women who had had face-lifts and those who were correctly made up.

There are new and effective methods available to us to revitalize our appearance. You might benefit by looking into them before deciding on surgery. One is a professional corrective technique for diminishing wrinkles as well as other unwelcome factors. Another is a new technique of redesigning your face with properly selected makeup to bring out its hidden beauty. Still another includes some special cosmetics adapted to the mature skin. I will explain them all.

### Complexion Make-over

There are now available a number of special, professional skin correction centers throughout the U.S., including Hawaii, and in Canada too. They feature a remarkable technique, developed by Jerry O'Neal, registered nurse and skin therapist. She is a frequent guest on radio and TV, and you may have seen or already heard of her.

The method, known as the Jeneal Treatment, is being increasingly recognized by physicians and other health professionals as a means of removing skin problems that are not considered diseases. Jeneal technicians are meticulously trained to correct or diminish such cosmetic disorders as wrinkles, large pores, stretch marks, acne-type conditions, pitting and scarring, and unwanted hair as well. Also, clients are instructed how to maintain beautiful skin at home during and following treatment.

I have seen before-and-after photos showing impressive results. Both men and women, along with health practitioners, express delight and full satisfaction with the Jeneal correction of skin disturbances or disfigurements that were considered beyond help.

If you are interested, you may write to Jeneal International Headquarters, 2721 Hillcroft, Houston, Texas 77027, for detailed information and the location of established centers. Also, Mrs. O'Neal will personally train qualified technicians who may want to provide this unique service in or near your community.

### New Miracle Makeup

The new miracle procedure I am about to describe is an exclusive for its presentation in this book, the first publication to announce this flattering, unusual technique. The method *redesigns* faces through makeup alone, diminishes wrinkles and flaws, bringing out beauty or good looks you may never have realized you had.

Ideally, it should be first applied by an expert, who can then show you your correct colors and other makeup products necessary, plus the know-how to do it yourself. Many beauty parlors have this service and the necessary cosmetics. Plans are also under way to help you by mail if you cannot find a salon that teaches this method to its clients.

The technique uses unique cosmetics called *Ambiage* (pronounced ahm-bia-zhe) and is the brainchild of Robert Marc, who has been one of Hollywood's leading makeup artists. He has founded Romarc Cosmetics Ltd., an institute for redesigning faces by skilled technicians, including his wife Aea (pronounced ee-a), who bring forth amazed "Oh's and Ah's" from clients using their method of facial design, which can create the illusion of a face-lift. I know, because it happened to me and others whose tranformation I have witnessed.

For more information write to Romarc Cosmetics Ltd., 6325 DeSoto Avenue, Woodland Hills, California 91367.

### Helpful, Effective Cosmetics for Mature Skins

Thanks to the new law that cosmetics must state ingredients on their labels, many previously unsuspected causes of allergies can be avoided. (It has been actually proved that what you apply to your skin can penetrate into your body and be later measured in your blood!)

The public can use all the help it can get in avoiding dangerous chemicals not only in foods but in cosmetics. Just to give you an idea of what can happen, these examples occur to me, all in connection with eye makeup. In some cases fiber-glass particles are added to mascara to give the illusion of longer lashes. What is to prevent these tiny fibers from becoming embedded in your eyes? I have heard that certain roll-on mascaras may also be dangerous on account of eye-irritating ingredients. Another example is that of an originally safe food product, a dietary protein, which was added to an eyelash grower. The original manufacturer sold his company, along with the cosmetic formulas, to new owners, who promptly added formaldehyde to the eyelash grower! The *Merck Index*, the "bible" on drugs and chemicals, states that formaldehyde is used as a disinfectant in buildings to kill flies and other insects, as well as in certain chemical processes to *harden* or render gelatine insoluble. (Gelatine is a protein; so is the eye. Who wants formaldehyde in *anything* that can invade the eye and irritate or make it hard?)

Other dangers apply to other cosmetics. That is not to say that these dangers might happen to everyone, but why take a chance? The unfortunate part about the new cosmetic labeling law is that some ingredients with long names may sound horrendous, but are relatively safe and essential to a formula's effectiveness, while others sound innocent, but under certain circumstances may be exceedingly dangerous. This means that the public—that is, you and I—*do not know* the difference between good and bad ingredients. If you are in any doubt, ask your library to show you Ruth Winter's book, *A Consumer's Dictionary of Cosmetic Ingredients*. (The paperback edition is published by Crown Publishers.) This book tells the *truth* about the effects of ingredients in cosmetics.

The reason I have mentioned the possible dangers of some cosmetics is to explain why the list that follows

is chosen only from those I have thoroughly researched and that are considered safe for the average
person. Even so, since allergies vary on a person-to-
person basis, this is no guarantee that you can be immune to everything. Products on which others may
thrive sometimes upset me or my friends, just as most
people can eat strawberries, whereas others dare not
eat them because of an allergic reaction. Even so, I am
proud to introduce to you the following skin and hair
products, which are as safe as I can find (I have
checked them with many chemists), and I recommend
them for that reason. Or, if you have already found a
product that agrees with your skin and body, by all
means treasure it.

## Skin Products

One company I have found trustworthy imports or
manufactures reliable cosmetics (both for skin improvement and makeup) made especially for Senior
skins. This company has pictures showing people of
various ages whose skins have found these products
beneficial. The company also manufactures skin products for men. It is called Reviva Labs (pronounced *Re-
veeva*), and is located at 24 E. Redman Ave., Haddonfield, New Jersey 08033. Stephen Strassler, presi-
dent of this company, really *cares* about your skin
problems. If Reviva products are not already in your
health stores, write, or ask the store to write, to Reviva Labs.

Among the most popular products from this company is its *Light Skin Peel*. This product, used once
weekly, safely and gently removes all dead surface

skin cells, and not only leaves your skin glowing, but because the pores have been freed of debris, they can better assimilate nourishing creams and lotions. Mr. Strassler says of this light skin peel: "It isn't the fountain of youth or the cure for all skin problems, but many users swear we're getting close."

Reviva also has some delightful cleansers, including a cleansing milk and a cleansing emulsion, both for sensitive as well as Senior skins. And now that Placenta is in the limelight, since the announcement that the Russians are using it to retard aging, Reviva has not been asleep at the switch. They have long had a mask featuring Placenta, which many of us use not only as a masque but also as a day or night cream, we like it so well.

And I cannot leave Reviva without mentioning their makeup items. Seniors must be careful to use only the minimum amount of makeup, as all screen and stage stars will tell you. Too much makeup, even some foundations lavishly applied, make you look older. But the colors of Reviva foundations (which are sheer) and blushers are delightful and flattering. Linda Clark reminds me to mention their lovely muted shades of lipsticks, which are in muted soft shades and safe. She prefers Reviva lipsticks to all others, she says.

Best of all, which is a special service from Reviva, are kits containing small sizes of cosmetics (cleansers, masques, and treatment creams) chosen especially for each age and skin category so that you may try before you buy larger amounts. If you are like me, your shelves are stacked with discarded cosmetics you found disappointing. I, who am a cosmetic guinea pig, trying them as fast as they appear on the market, often cannot find room in my refrigerator for food—it is so crowded with cosmetics! (Sample kits can prevent this for you.) Reviva has many other delightful products from which to choose.

There is a new cosmetic company called Mill Creek Natural Products, with headquarters in Rolling Hills, California, and their products are available in health stores. These products are made of *really* natural, safe ingredients. In addition to skin products, there are also some hair products (mentioned later under hair). And they have a *superb* roll-on deodorant that contains no poisonous chemicals at all, a very rare find these days.

Another face cream is the genuine Dr. Benjamin S. Frank, M.D.'s *Nutrient Cream*, formulated by Dr. Frank to smooth away wrinkles. Some people achieve excellent results with this cream, rich in RNA. Others, with dry skin or who live in dry climates, find it necessary to add a few drops of water or their favorite moisturizer on top of the cream after applying it to the face. This Dr. Frank Nutrient Cream is available from The Prime of Life, Inc., P.O. Box 5107, FDR Station, New York, N.Y. 10022. You can write for information.

If you want a nice, heavy, yellow, ointment-type healing cream for severe dryness, wrinkling, and chapping, there is an excellent formula called *Tocophoderm,* which contains natural vitamins A and E and natural oils as well as lecithin. This product is quickly absorbed. Linda Clark tells me that members of her family consider this cream very effective. It is made by Nutri-Dyn, the same company that manufactures those glandular substances you have already read about.

One of my favorites is not a cream, but a powder-fine white clay called *Nevalite*. It is moistened with water and can be used for almost everything from a beautifying masque, to a moisturizer, or for relieving the irritation caused by poison oak or ivy. It is loaded with minerals, now known to be a help in prevention of aging. I would not be without it.

## *Hair*

The outdated description of hair as a "crowning glory" seems to have vanished for both men and women these days, due to air pollution, poor nutrition, stress, and other, undetected causes. There *are* ways to correct hair loss and other hair problems, as explained in Linda Clark's book *Secrets of Health and Beauty*, so I will not repeat them here. Hair growth can usually be induced, and I have seen it happen, so you do not need to depend upon a wig for the rest of your life, unless you wish.

I am more concerned with improving and beautifying the hair you already have, no matter how sparse or discouraging its present condition. I have seen amazing results take place with hair that was once considered hopeless by its owner and has today become truly a "crowning glory." Furthermore, these transformations were accomplished by products that are absolutely safe, whether a coloring, a permanent, or even a hair spray. First, let's talk about safe and beautiful hair coloring you can apply yourself in your own home.

Although many of us have known about, and warned against, some dangerous hair dyes for years, only recently has the FDA discovered and publicized the danger. We have learned that many illnesses, as well as allergies, rashes, and other unpleasant side effects, have been traced to unsafe hair dyes, due to dangerous chemicals they contain. Some people even develop suspicious, dark circles under their eyes as a result of continuous use of these questionable dyes (although this is not the only cause of dark circles, merely a clue in some cases to avoid using such poisons). With this explanation, it will come as no surprise to learn that I recommend only hair products that are *safe* as well as effective.

There is such a hair coloring product called *Vita Wave*, made from fruits, herbs, and vegetables. Stephan Molchan, of North Hollywood, California, the manufacturer, guarantees that his products contain no harsh or dangerous chemicals. The colors range from pale blonde to deep black (a no-no for most Seniors, as this is too harsh and aging for later years). Even safe bleaches available in this line may, for some very light shades, need some prebleaching with a Vita Wave hair lightener. Some consulting may help you get started either for this or other colors. Since you can order these products from Beauty Naturally, Inc., I am ready to help you with your problems on hair (as well as skin) if you wish to write me. (You will find my address at the end of this chapter.)

If you prefer professional, on-the-spot help, some beauty salons carry this same hair color product under the name *Vé Borné*. But many of us prefer to use these colorings in the privacy of our own home. Once you get the knack of using them, it is easy to do so as often as needed.

Vita Wave also has a safe do-it-yourself permanent,

guaranteed to be free of thioglycolic acid, a chemical that seems to generate many adverse reactions. This too is carried in some beauty salons under the name Vé Bonné.

If Vé Borné is not available in your salon, there is another safe permanent sold to beauty salons exclusively called *Nugania*. It is described like this: "A superb perm! No heat needed . . . no ammonia . . . wind with water only." And it is guaranteed not to harm the hair. The founder of this product and head of the company that supplies it is A. F. Willat, a remarkable scientist/inventor, now in his nineties and still in business.

Vita Wave also has a delightful hair spray made from fruits, herbs, and flowers. It is nonaerosol (avoiding the dangers of propellants) and provides a mist free of the usual harsh ingredients found in other sprays and is expelled by a plunger. It is gradually absorbed into the hair to add body. It also brushes or combs out easily, is water soluble (not gummy). For all these reasons this spray is very popular.

Here are a few tips to keep in mind in hair-tinting. If you will look at a naturally colored head of hair, you will see that there are many different shades instead of a flat, solid color—a giveaway that hair has been dyed. One way to achieve the natural look is by applying the tint, in some areas, on dry rather than damp hair.

If salons do not carry these safe products, keep insisting until they do! Do not accept something "just as good" (in their opinion).

Now for other hair-beautifying products. There are some really dramatic helps here.

*Chenti Panthenol products.*

Panthenol is actually a provitamin, meaning that when it is used on the skin or hair it becomes pantothenic acid, or vitamin B-5. Laboratory tests show actual photographs of a damaged, frizzled, frayed, or split strand of hair before and after the application of Panthenol. Almost immediately the hair is repaired, smooth, and develops more strength and body.

The medical profession has used Panthenol for treating hair and skin problems for years, but only recently has the beauty industry adopted it. I prefer the Chenti brand because it contains more of this remarkable substance than most other brands, which, though listing Panthenol on the label, may contain only a "drop in the bucket," so to speak, compared to the greater amount found in Chenti products.

Chenti Panthenol products include a shampoo and an amino acid Panthenol Treatment, a lotion applied after rinsing the hair to repair and give it body. The whole line is terrific!

There are also some Chenti skin products containing vitamins A,D, and E that are very popular, including a cream and a body lotion often used on the face.

If you do not find Chenti products at your health store, write to Beauty Naturally.

Panthenol has also been used by another company to strengthen nails in a surprisingly short time. If you have nail problems, write me.

Keratin protein is another hair strengthener. Mill Creek Laboratories, mentioned earlier, make these hair products available exclusively for health stores. And don't forget that fabulous deodorant from Mill

Creek Laboratories. This is also available from Beauty Naturally.

So now you see that it is possible to appear at your best, or even better than best, regardless of your age. With these bounties I have described, you can do it yourself at home with very little money and lots of satisfaction.

If you need help with your hair or skin problems or wish to keep up with new discoveries, just write to Betty Franklin, Beauty Naturally, Inc., Box 426, Fairfax, California 94930. Please remember to include a large, business-size self-addressed, stamped envelope.

REFERENCES
(See *Bibliography* for fuller details.)

1. Linda Clark, *Face Improvement Through Exercise and Nutrition.*
2. Senta Maria Rungé, *Face Lifting by Exercise.*

# 18

## Your Rejuvenation Blueprint

**A SUMMARY**

1. You need to rebuild your body by rebuilding your cells. This is done mainly by feeding your cells the best fuel available. Although vitamins and minerals are important, you need, first and foremost, the right kind of food. Introduce the high-powered foods, mentioned in Chapter 11, gradually into your diet. This provides your health foundation. Then add vitamin/mineral supplements as needed. Read *Know Your Nutrition* to learn which ones they are. Be sure to eat plenty of raw foods and sprouts. Eat less, chew more.

Good health does not come instantly, but you will notice it on a good day now and then after you embark on your new program. The good days gradually increase until they are the rule, not the exception.

2. Find the exercise that appeals to you and do it daily. Be sure to do your breathing exercises too.

3. Watch your thinking. Set up your blueprint according to how you want to feel, look, and act. Follow through, no matter what temptation arises, until good thinking becomes a habit.

4. Radiate love to everyone, and your inner beauty (or handsomeness, if you are a man) will take care of itself.

5. Improve your appearance. You have been given some of the ways to do this in Chapter 17.

Meanwhile, don't stoop when you stand, sit, or walk. Stand tall like royalty! The best exercise I know for becoming erect is the one I have often told about the young girl who had miserable posture, as well as a spinal curvature. She invented this exercise, which not only led to her being used as a model on the Liberty quarter (at the beginning of World War I), but overcame her spinal curvature, as confirmed by a physician. Here are the directions for the exercise:

Put your hands behind your back, arms straight, hands back to back. Interlace the backs of the fingers of both hands. Now twist your thumbs, first toward your spine, then away from it. Repeat often. It straightens your spine, raises your chest, and pulls in your stomach.

When you walk, do not give away your age by shuffling. Stride, swinging your legs from your hips, your arms from the shoulders.

*You can't look well if you don't feel well.* As reported in Richard Passwater's book, *Supernutrition*, a five-year study of seven thousand California residents was conducted by researchers at the University of California. "They studied seven health habits and found that people who get adequate sleep, eat breakfast, stay lean, avoid empty calorie snacks (pastries, soda pop, candy, cookies), don't smoke, exercise regularly, and either don't drink or take very little alcohol are rewarded with superior health. . . . Those who followed all the good practices were in better health at every age than those who only followed one or few." In other words, you must program your rejuvenation, not leave it to chance.

Another example: One woman, a great-grandmother, refused to act her age. Instead of knitting or gossiping, she took up basketball, swimming, and bowling. Adding good nutrition and good thinking to such a program will make you a winner!

So influence the years you live, don't let the years you live influence you.

And if anyone asks you how you are, don't whine, "Pretty well." Stand up straight, look the other person straight in the eye, and even if you temporarily feel like falling over, say firmly, "FINE!" Like a strong, instead of a fishy, handshake, that should get the message across to everybody, including your subconscious, that whatever your age, you mean success.

Appoint yourself a committee of one to start reversing the poor image of Seniors. Help us all to make the most of our potential so that we can be proud of ourselves and our group. *Start Now.*

I hope the information in this book will add happy years to your life. Forget your age and make the most of your years, which should be the best part of your life. Make them so!

# 19

## Rejuvenation
## From Tibet

I HAVE SAVED the most exciting method of rejuvenation for the last. In 1975 I was introduced to a chemical engineer. He knew of my work and told me he had come across a method of rejuvenation that might interest me. He sent me a small booklet called *The Five Rites of Rejuvenation.*[1] This booklet contains an almost incredible story.

It concerns an elderly, retired British army colonel who looked, felt, and acted old. When he had been stationed in India, some natives had told him of a lamasery, where the lamas had discovered the secret of youth. In this group there were no people who looked, felt, or acted old.

After a long, exhaustive search he finally found the group and asked to be taught the technique. When he first arrived, he was called "The Ancient One." But after a month on the technique he no longer looked ancient. When he first saw himself in a mirror, he couldn't believe the change, and when he returned to England no one recognized him—except those who thought he was his son!

The colonel explained the method to a friend, telling him it had been kept secret for centuries. The technique he was taught is explained in the booklet, and I shall give it here.

> The body has seven magnetic centers, called vortexes. In a healthy body they revolve at great speed; when they slow down, ill health, old age, senility appear.
>
> These vortexes are located as follows: two in the brain; one at the base of the throat; one in the right side above the waist line; one in the reproductive anatomy; and one in each knee.
>
> These spinning centers of activity extend beyond the flesh in the healthy individual, but not in the old, weak, or senile person. The quickest way to regain health, youth, and vitality is to start these magnetic centers spinning again.
>
> There are five exercises. Any one will be helpful, but all five are required to get glowing results. The lamas call them Rites, instead of exercises.

After the colonel achieved his own rejuvenation in India, he returned to England and started small classes in which he taught the Rites. He refused to enroll any person under fifty years old. Every single student reported improvement. One of them, a man close to seventy-five, made especially remarkable progress.

The five Rites are practiced once each three times daily to start, and increased to twenty-one times daily.

All five Rites require only a few minutes. One day a week can be missed, but no more. The booklet states that improvement continues even after two years, when a still more pronounced change in appearance and condition is possible.

Both men and women can do them. My chemical engineer acquaintance told me he had practiced them himself for two years. I had never seen him before, but at sixty he looks closer to forty-five. Another man wrote me that he had practiced the Rites for six years with nothing but highly satisfactory results, although he did indicate that good nutrition was also necessary. This man now practices the Rites only ten times a day. If you cannot keep up the twenty-one times, settle for as many as seem comfortable for you.

The Rites are not really difficult, although you have to get used to some of them. Stiffness may interfere initially, but this soon passes. The whirling exercise, should be taken carefully at first. If you get dizzy, STOP, sit down, and wait until the next session to try it again. Eventually you will find that the longer you work at the Rites, the easier they become.

In the pages that follow I shall give, with the permission of the publisher, a description of the five Rites, accompanied by an illustration of each. However, I do suggest that you order a copy of the booklet without delay, to get the full, fascinating story (I have told only a portion of it). It costs only $2.50, and I hope, having introduced it to the public, the supply lasts. You may order *The Five Rites of Rejuvenation* from Borderland Sciences Research Foundation, P.O. Box 548, Vista, Calif. 92083. (Californians, please add tax.)

THE RITES

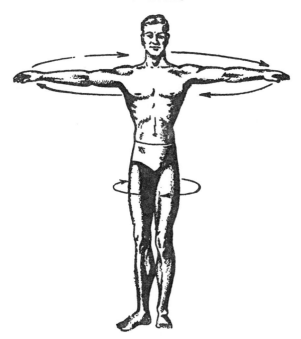

**Rite No. 1**

Stand erect, arms outstretched, horizontal with the shoulders. Now turn around in a *clockwise direction* only. Fasten your eyes on a starting point and count rotations as you return to this spot. At first, practice this Rite only to the point of slight dizziness. As time passes and your vortexes revolve more rapidly, you will be able to repeat the Rite more often with less discomfort. Take it easy.

Lie full length on the floor. Place your arms, palms flat on the floor, alongside your hips. Raise your feet until your legs are straight up. If possible, let them extend lightly beyond your head, but do not bend your knees. Then slowly lower your legs to the floor, relax and repeat.

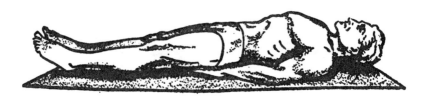

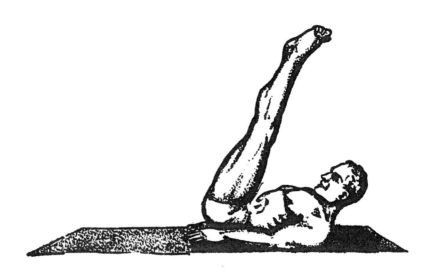

## Rite No. 2

One of the lamas found when he began this exercise that he was so old, weak, and decrepit he could not possibly lift both legs. With bent knees at first, he lifted his thighs, letting his feet hang down. Little by little he could straighten his legs. By the end of the third month he could lift them straight up with ease.

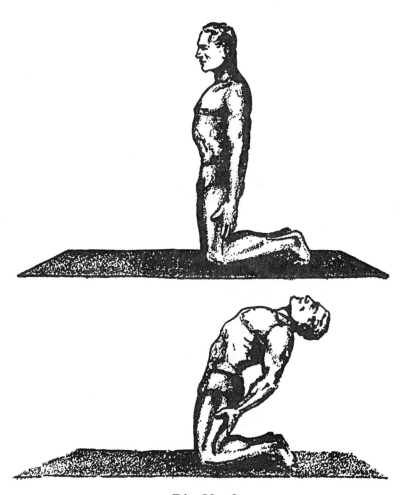

## Rite No. 3

Kneel on the floor, place your hands on your thighs and lean as far forward as possible, with your chin resting on your chest.

Now lean backward as far as possible, also leaning the head backward as far as it will go.

Bring your head upright, body straight, to starting position. Repeat the Rite.

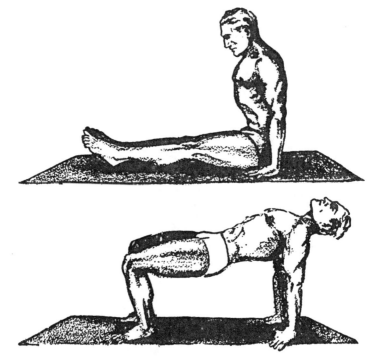

### Rite No. 4

This seems hard at first, but after a week becomes surprisingly easy. Sit on the floor, feet and legs outstretched in front of you. Place your hands palms down, arms straight directly under your shoulders, against your body. Put your head or chin on your chest.

Now bend your knees, feet flat on the floor, and raise your body until it makes a table. Let your head drop gently backward as far as it will go. Return to a sitting position, then repeat. If you cannot get the "feel" of it, do not become discouraged. You might lie on a low box at first until you can eventually push your body to a table position without a prop.

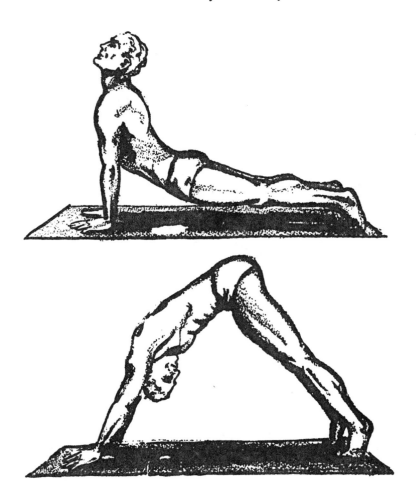

## Rite No. 5

Place your hands, palms down, on the floor. Kneel on your knees, and then stretch your body upward until your hips are as high as possible. Head should be down and forward.

Slowly lower your hips until your body sags. Let your head bend back as far as possible. Return to a knee position and repeat.

Some Rites are harder for some, whereas others are harder for others. Rites No. 4 and 5 are more difficult for most people. But do the ones you can, and try the others until you become proficient in all. Sooner or later your muscles will become strong, and you will be able to do them all with ease.

These Rites can be practiced morning or night, or both. But because they are stimulating, morning might be best.

Three times a day for the first week is recommended. Then increase them by two a day until you are doing twenty-one a day, which will be the beginning of the tenth week.

If you cannot do the whirling Rite, number one, the same number of times as the others, do it only as many times as you can without getting too dizzy. Eventually you will be able to do it the same number of times as the others. If you have had any injury or operation, wait until you are well before beginning them (ask your doctor).

These illustrations and directions will give you the necessary information for their use. More complete directions appear in the booklet. Adjust them to your own ability to perform them. Continuous use brings results.

**REFERENCES**

(See *Bibliography* for fuller details.)

1. Peter Kelder, *The Five Rites of Rejuvenation.*

# Postscript:
# If You Need Help

If after reading this book, you have further questions from time to time, please do not write to Linda Clark personally, as, due to her crowded schedule, she cannot correspond with readers. Instead, send your questions to Linda Clark's column, "Extend Your Lifeline," published monthly in a newsletter called *Good Healthkeeping,* which includes helpful information for all ages from outstanding writers knowledgeable in the field of health, aging, beauty, and other related subjects.

Although the subscription price of *Good Healthkeeping* is far less than that of similar publications, if you prefer you may subscribe jointly with other Seniors and share the cost and the information in the newsletter. However, please send only one name and address for each subscription.

Questions are, of course, welcome from all. When you mail in your query, you will be sent the first issue of *Good Healthkeeping* free with information about subscription rates.

Address:

*Good Healthkeeping*
Price-Pottenger Nutrition Foundation
P.O. Box 2614
La Mesa, Calif. 92041

Questions should be marked: Attention, Linda Clark's column "Extend Your Lifeline." Please allow two months for answers to your questions—the usual time lapse for all magazines.

# Suggested Reading

Benet, Sula, *How to Live to be 100*. New York: Dial Press, 1976

Blaine, Tom R., *Goodbye Allergies*. New York: Kensington Publishing Corp.

Bloodsworth, Venice, M.D., *Key to Yourself*. (Available from Scrivener & Co., Publishers, 6007 Barton Avenue, Los Angeles, Calif. 90038.)

Bock, Raymond F., M.D., *Vitamin E: Key to Youthful Longevity*. Hicksville, N.Y.: Exposition Press, Inc.

Carter, Mildred, *Helping Yourself to Foot Reflexology*. West Nyack, N.Y.: Parker Publishing Company

Chang, Stephen T., with Rick Miller, *The Book of Internal Exercises*. San Francisco, Calif.: Strawberry Hill Press, 1977

Chapman, J.B., M.D., edited by Cogswell, J.W., M.D., *Dr. Schuessler's Biochemistry*. London: New Era Laboratories Ltd. (Available in the United States from Standard Homeopathic Pharmacy, P.O. Box 61067, Los Angeles, Calif. 90061.)

Cheng Man-ching, and Smith, Robert W., *T'ai Chi*. Rutland, Vermont: Charles Tuttle Company

Christopher, John R., M.D., *Rejuvenation through Elimination.* (Booklet available from The Herb Shop, Box 352, Provo, Utah 84601.)

Clark, Linda, *Be Slim and Healthy.* New Canaan, Conn.: Keats Publishing Company, 1972

——————, *Color Therapy.* Old Greenwich, Conn.: The Devin-Adair Company, 1975; New York: Pocket Books, 1978, paperback

——————, *Face Improvement through Exercise and Nutrition.* New Canaan, Conn.: Keats Publishing Company

——————, *A Handbook of Natural Remedies for Common Ailments.* Old Greenwich, Conn.: The Devin-Adair Company, 1976; New York: Pocket Books, 1978, paperback

——————, *Know Your Nutrition.* New Canaan, Conn.: Keats Publishing Company, 1973

——————, *Secrets of Health and Beauty.* Old Greenwich, Conn.: The Devin-Adair Company, 1969; New York: Pyramid Books, 1971, paperback

——————, *Stay Young Longer.* New York: Pyramid Books, 1968, paperback

——————, *The Best of Linda Clark* (an anthology). New Canaan, Conn.: Keats Publishing Company, 1976

——————, with Karen Kelly, *Beauty Questions and Answers.* New York: Pyramid Books, 1977

——————, with Yvonne Martine, *Health, Youth and Beauty through Color Breathing.* Millbrae, Calif.: Celestial Arts; *also* New York: Berkely. Both paperbacks

Cordy, Don, *The Protein Book.* Healdsburg, Calif.: Naturegraph Publishers, Inc.

*Course in Miracles, A,* 3 vols. New York: Foundation for Inner Peace (1 West 81st Street, New York, N.Y. 10024)

Davis, Adelle, *Let's Eat Right to Keep Fit.* New York: New American Library, Signet paperback

Delaney, Walter, *Ultra Psychonics*. West Nyack, N.Y.: Parker Publishing Company, 1975

Dextreit, Raymond, *Our Earth, Our Cure*. (English publication available from Swan Publishing Company, P.O. Box 170, Brooklyn, N.Y. 11223.)

Ellis, John M., M.D., with Presley, James, *B6, The Doctor's Report*. New York: Harper and Row, 1973

Franklyn, Robert Alan, M.D., *Shiatsu—60 Minutes to Facial Beauty*. (Available from Doctor Beauty, Inc., Publications, 8760 Sunset Boulevard, Los Angeles, Calif. 90067.)

Halsell, Grace, *Los Viejos, Secrets of Long Life from the Sacred Valley*. Emmaus, Pa.: Rodale Press, 1976

Houston, F.M., *The Healing Benefits of Acupressure*. New Canaan, Conn.: Keats Publishing Company

Howell, Edward, M.D., "The Status of Food Enzymes in Digestion and Metabolism," *Chemical Abstracts and Biological Abstracts*, 1946

Hungerford, Mary Jane, "Nutritional Factors in Common Behavior Problems," *Journal of Applied Nutrition*, Vol. 27, No. 4, Winter 1975

Jensen, Bernard, *World Keys to Health and Long Life*. Escondido, Calif.: Omni Publishers

Kaye, Anna, with Don C. Matchan, *Mirror of the Body*. San Francisco, Calif.: Strawberry Hill Press, 1977

Kelder, Peter, *The Five Rites of Rejuvenation*. (Available from The Borderland Sciences, Research Foundation, Box 548, Vista, Calif. 92083.)

Kübler-Ross, Elisabeth, *On Death and Dying*. New York: Macmillan, 1969, hardcover and paperback
——————, *Death, The Final Stage of Growth*. Englewood Cliffs, N.J.: Prentice-Hall, 1975

Kugler, Hans J., *Slowing Down the Aging Process*. New York: Pyramid Books, 1975, paperback

——————, *Seven Keys to a Longer Life.* New York: Stein & Day, 1977

Leonard, Jon N., Hofer, J.L., Pritikin, N., *Live Longer Now.* New York: Grosset & Dunlap, 1974

Matchan, Don C., *We Mind If You Smoke.* New York: Pyramid, 1977

Martin, Wayne, *Medical Heroes and Heretics.* Old Greenwich, Conn.: The Devin-Adair Company, 1977

Moody, Raymond A., Jr., M.D., *Life After Life.* New York: Mockingbird Books, 1975; New York, Bantam Books, 1976, paperback

Morrison, Lester M., M.D., *The Low-Fat Way to Health and Longer Life.* Englewood Cliffs, N.J.: Prentice-Hall, 1958

Nittler, Alan H., M.D., *A New Breed of Doctor.* New York: Pyramid Books, 1974, paperback

Norton, Suza, *Yoga for People Over 50.* Old Greenwich, Conn.: The Devin-Adair Company, 1977, paperback edition available

Passwater, Richard A., *Supernutrition.* New York: Dial Press, 1975

——————, *Supernutrition for Healthy Hearts.* New York:Dial Press, 1977

Popov, Ivan, M.D., *Stay Young.* New York: Grosset & Dunlap, 1975

Rungé, Senta Maria, *Face Lifting by Exercise.* (Available from P.O. Box 39523, Los Angeles, Calif. 90039.)

Silva, José, and Miele, Philip, *The Silva Mind Control Method.* New York: Simon and Schuster, 1977

Smith, Robert Kimmel, *Sadie Shapiro's Knitting Book.* New York: Fawcett Publications, 1973, paperback (a rollicking, funny short novel about an over-70 "Senior" who keeps herself and others moving)

——————, *Sadie Shapiro in Miami.* New York: Simon and Schuster, 1977 (a sequel in which Sadie, practically single-handed, changes the Senior world)

Stearn, Jess, *The Power of Alpha Thinking.* New York: New American Library, a Signet paperback

Stephenson, James R., M.D., *A Doctor's Guide to Helping Yourself with Homeopathic Remedies.* West Nyack, N.Y.: Parker Publishing Company

Williams, Roger J., *Biochemical Individuality.* New York: Wiley, 1956; now available in paperback from the University of Texas Press

——————, *Nutrition Against Disease.* New York: Pitman Publishing Corporation, 1971; New York, Bantam Books, 1973, paperback

——————, *You Are Extraordinary.* New York: Random House, 1967

Winter, Ruth, *A Consumer's Dictionary of Cosmetic Ingredients.* New York: Crown Publishers

# PRODUCT LIST

Try your health store for the following products. If they do not have them, use the address indicated beside the product (or products) you want. For information about all others write to: Beauty Naturally, Inc., P.O. Box 426, Fairfax, California 94030. Please include a stamped, long (business-size), self-addressed envelope with your request, or a loose stamp.

*Ambiage*, Romarc Cosmetics Ltd., 6325 DeSoto Avenue, Woodland Hills, Calif. 91367

*Bio-Strath* tablets (contain RNA and herbs), Beauty Naturally, Inc.

*Birkenstock* sandals, 1016 B Street, San Rafael, Calif. 94901, or Beauty Naturally, Inc.

*Calms Forté* (cell salts and herbs) and *Nerve Tonic* tablets, Standard Homeopathic Pharmacy, Box 61067, Los Angeles, Calif. 90061

*Dr. Frank's Nutrient Cream*, The Prime of Life, Inc., P.O. Box 5107, FDR Station, New York, N.Y. 10022

*Green Clay*, The Three Sheaves Company, 100 Varick

Street, New York, N.Y. 10013. Write for catalog with prices.

*Ipsab* (for gums). Beauty Naturally, Inc.

*Jeneal Treatment* (for skin correction). Beauty salons or write to Jeneal, 2721 Hillcroft, Houston, Texas 77027

*Kyolic* Garlic. Available at most health stores

*Lachle's Original High Energy Multi-Purpose Food* (protein powder). Health stores or Beauty Naturally, Inc.

*Malabar glandular protein powder.* Available at most health stores or Beauty Naturally, Inc., or write to Malabar Cor-ron Products, Box 1021, Pacific Palisades, Calif. 90272

*Milk Digestant*, Malabar Cor-ron Products, Box 1021, Pacific Palisades, Calif. 90272, or health stores and Beauty Naturally, Inc.

*Minerals 72.* Write to Beauty Naturally, Inc.

*Nerve Tonic* tablets (homeopathic cell salts). Standard Homeopathic Pharmacy, Box 61067, Los Angeles, Calif. 90061

*Nutri-Dyn* raw gland concentrates. Nutri-Dyn Products Corp., 5705 Howard Street, Niles, Ill. 60648, or ask for *Search* products at health stores. (Nutri-Dyn has another office in Florida, where Caroline Cropp is located. Its address is: Nutri-Dyn American Distributors, 2320 S.W. 60th Way, Hollywood, Florida 33023.)

*Periwinkle Extract*, Bio-Botanica, 2 Willow Park, Farmingdale, N.Y. 11735. (In ordering specify "*Vinca major* and *Vinca minor.*)

*Protomorphogens* (glandular and organ extracts in tablet form). Standard Process Laboratories, Inc. (division of Vitamin Products Company), 2023 W. Wisconsin Avenue, Milwaukee, Wisconsin 53201. These are available *only* through doctors, although the doctor may be an M.D., D.O., D.C., even a D.D.S. You should have your doctor write for the nearest branch office of this company in your area.

*Reviva* skin products and cosmetics, Reviva Labs, E. Redman Avenue, Haddonfield, New Jersey 08033

*Sundancer Exerciser.* Write to Olympus Distributing Corporation, 180 North 200 East, St. George, Utah 84770, requesting information on distributors in your area.

Vita Herbs, Inc., 1348 Baur Blvd., Warson Road, Industrial Park, St. Louis, Mo. 63132. These are excellent products combining vitamins and herbs. Write for catalogue. For choosing products for specific ailments, ask your doctor to order this information for you. Letters from patients cannot be answered.

*Vita Wave* hair products (for safe coloring and permanents). Health stores or Beauty Naturally, Inc.

*Zell Oxygen.* Can be ordered from Bio-Nutritional Products, P.O. Box 1494, FDR Station, New York, N.Y. 10022

# INDEX

# Notes for Your
# Rejuvenation Program